Instructor's Guide

by

Barbara A. Gylys, MEd, CMA-A

to accompany

Computer Applications for the Medical Office: Patriot Medical®
second edition

by

Barbara A. Gylys, MEd, CMA-A

 F. A. Davis Company • Philadelphia

F. A. Davis Company
1915 Arch Street
Philadelphia, PA 19103

Last digit indicates print number: 10 9 8 7 6 5 4 3 2 1

Printed in the United States of America

ISBN 0-8036-0083-6

CONTENTS

THIS INSTALLATION REQUIRES THE EXPERTISE OF A COMPUTER TECHNICIAN

HARD DRIVE DOCUMENTATION

System Requirements

- IBM or compatible PC with at least 4 Mb RAM
- one 5.25-inch or 3.5-inch high density disk drive
- DotMatrix or Laser printer

Program Installation

Before you can run the ***Patriot Medical® (PM),*** the two program disks must be installed on your hard disk. It is recommended that you make a back-up copy of both disks before installing the program. The installation procedure decompresses and copies files from the two program disks onto your hard disk to create the *PM* program. Use the back-up copy and follow the instructions below to install the two program disks.

Note: If using Windows, exit the Windows environment prior to starting this procedure.

1. Create a *Patriot* directory on your hard drive for the software program.

> - At the C-prompt (C:\>) type:
>
>   MD \PATRIOT (Press ENTER)
>   CD \PATRIOT (Press ENTER)

2. Copy the contents of ***Patriot Medical® Student Version Program*** disk to the directory on your hard drive.

> - Put Disk1 in drive A.
> - At the C-prompt type:
>
>   COPY A: *.* (Press ENTER)

3. At the *Patriot* directory prompt, type **INSTALL**, and press Enter. The program will begin to extract the program files .

4. Copy the contents of ***Patriot Medical®, Fox Pro 2.0 Extended Runtime*** disk to the *Patriot* directory.

> - Put Disk 2 in drive A.
> - At the C-prompt type:
>
>   COPY A: *.* (Press ENTER)

5. At the *Patriot* directory prompt, type **FOXRTX**, and press Enter. The program will begin to extract the *FoxPro* runtime files.

6. At the *Patriot* directory prompt, type **STUINST**, and press Enter. The *Patriot Medical Installation Procedure* screen will display on your monitor.

7. Press Enter at the highlighted *Student Setup* option. Either accept the path where the program files are located by pressing Enter or enter your path and press Enter.

8. When you are finished, return to the *Patriot Medical Installation Procedure* screen. Then, press the hot key R to return to the *Patriot* directory.

Edit the Config.Sys File:

9. In your CONFIG.SYS file, set the buffers to equal 40 and files to equal 100.

> Note: You will need a text-editor program to change the CONFIG.SYS file. If you are not familiar with text-editor programs, you should have someone knowledgeable in this area do this for you.

Installation Verification of Patriot Software

1. To verify that the software is installed correctly, boot up your system (Note: remove all diskettes from your drives before re-booting. Then, place the *Patriot Medical® Student Version Data Disk* in your drive

2. At the C-prompt (if you are in Windows you must exit Windows first) type **cd\patriot**.

3. At the *Patriot* directory prompt, type **student**. Use *PM* as a password. At the Main Menu opening screen, scroll to the Master Files Menu and access some of the files. When you are finished, scroll to Quit at the Master Files Menu and sign off the PM program.

4. If you were able to complete the sign-on procedure, your installation is complete. If you encounter any error messages while trying to run *PM,* refer to the *Trouble Shooting Guide* in the *Network Installation* section on page 3 for additional installation instructions.

NETWORK DOCUMENTATION

This program will not run **networked** on Windows '95. To run the program in Windows '95, restart in MS DOS mode.

The network installation for the PM software is written and tested on the Novell Network System. The installation requires the expertise of a network specialist. The same documentation principles apply when installing the software on other network operating systems.

For the network, Novell Network is the operating system of choice. Past experiences with Lantastic/non-dedicated servers have proven inadequate for FoxPro.

Multi-User Network System Requirements

Multi-user network environment which comprises of a stand alone/dedicated server and numerous workstations.

Suggested Server: Minimum 486 DX2 66Mhz PC, Novell Network Operating Software, Windows, etc. 16mb RAM, PCI Local Bus; 540mb of hard disk space.

Recommended Server: 486DX4 100 MHz or a Pentium-based machine with 32mb RAM. running Novell Neware o/s.

Suggested Workstation: 486DX2 50mhx workstation with 8mb RAM.

Recommended Workstation: 486DX2 66 MHz workstations with 16mb RAM.

Please note that running on a 386 or less and 8 mbRAM on the server and workstations (8mb RAM and 4mb RAM respectively), speed will be sacrificed and the program will run slow, particularly when the students use the Appointment Scheduler. The optimum set up would accommodate the transition to MS Windows 95 and future versions of PM.

The FoxPro Extended Runtime version can take advantage of extended memory or extended memory made to act like expanded memory, but it cannot mix and match the two. If only part of your extended memory is acting like expanded, the extended version will only use the memory that is acting like expanded memory.

To improve the performance of PM, we recommend that you load your Terminate and Stay Resident (TSRs) programs high.

Other Hardware

Dot matrix or laser printers. If printing jobs are channeled to a shared printer via the network, the user will probably have to exit the application before the print is released to the printer. Instructor's should be advised to inform their students of the printing procedure, preferably with a handout and oral directions.

HARD DRIVE AND NETWORK TROUBLE SHOOTING GUIDE

Hard Drive

The CONFIG.SYS file is not a FoxPro file. It's a file that is used by the computer's operating system to establish the working environment. Because FoxPro interacts with this environment, you must be sure that certain settings are properly established. BUFFERS= and FILES= are CONFIG.SYS statements of immediate importance to FoxPro. If these settings are not set properly, you will experience some error messages. Verify that your config.sys file is set according to the following specifications:

```
Device=C:\DOS\HIMEM.SYS
Device=C:\DOS\EMM386.exe  4096 RAM
DOS=HIGH
Buffers=40
Files=100
```

When changes are made to the config.sys file, you must reboot the computer for the changes to take effect.

If the message **"TOO MANY FILES OPEN"** or **"File 'MERR' does not exist,"** displays on your monitor when you attempt to run the software, Patriot Medical® will not run because there are not enough file handles allocated to run the software.

Network

The **"TOO MANY FILES OPEN"** message may occur with Novell network users because the default value that Novell assigns to the file handles is 40. Certain operations in *PM* require more than 40 files to be opened at one time. To prevent this problem, set the file handles correctly before installing the *PM* application. If you are using Novell 2.1x or higher, do the following:

1. Add the following line to either the **shell.cfg** or **net.cfg** file: **file handles=75.**

2. If you don't have a **shell.cfg** or **net.cfg file**, create one using the DOS 5.0 edit command. Also, make sure that you enter a space between the words **files** and **handles.**

3. Novell 3.1x looks for **net.cfg** first, and then for **shell.cfg.** If there is no **net.cfg,** Novell only looks for **shell.cfg.**

4. You must place **shell.cfg/net.cfg** in the same directory where the **IPX** and **NET** Novell drivers reside. You must also load these drivers from that directory. Otherwise, **net.cfg** or **shell.cfg** will not be read. To find which directory Novell drivers reside in, check your **autoexec.bat** file.

Loading The Network Drivers

The following example shows the correct way to load the network drivers so that **shell.cfg/net.cfg** will be read correctly.

Correct Installation. You must perform the following actions for every computer on the network that uses PM.

```
F:>cd\novell
F:\novell>loadhigh ipx301
F:\novell>loadhigh netx
F:\novell>cd\
```

The following example shows an incorrect installation.

Incorrect Installation. The following method is incorrect because the user loads ipx and net from the Novell directory without actually being in the directory.

```
F:>loadhigh c:\novell\ipx301
F:>loadhigh c:\novell\netx
```

Insufficient Memory

This error will occur if you do not have enough Conventional Memory. This is the first 640K of memory on your computer. You should try and get as much of this a possible (minimum of 512K). You can increase the amount of conventional memory by loading TSR programs high.

TECHNICAL SUPPORT

Please contact F.A. Davis Technical Support at 888-FADAVIS (888-323-2847) if you require technical assistance.

OVERVIEW OF TEXTBOOK, INSTRUCTOR'S GUIDE, AND SOFTWARE

Computer Applications for the Medical Office: Patriot Medical®, *second edition,* is an interactive, competency-based approach to learning computerized management of a medical office. Students are guided through typical medical office administrative activities with the student version of Patriot Medical®, a widely utilized medical administrative software. The text and user-friendly software are designed to gradually introduce material of steadily increasing difficulty.

The learning package helps students develop medical office computer skills while progressing through various menus. They learn how to enter patient information, schedule appointments, complete the billing cycle, process insurance claims both on forms and electronically, and also perform numerous computer tasks. Students who learn Patriot Medical® will find that the software is similar to other medical office account management systems. Thus, within a very short period of time, they will be able to transfer their competence to any other system.

To teach the course more effectively, this comprehensive *Instructor's Guide* provides teachers with many supplementary items. Hopefully, it will help them to use their time in the most productive way, to the benefit of both teachers and students.

The two disks provided in each copy of the Instructor's Guide along with the student data disk in the textbook contain everything necessary for installing and running the Patriot Medical® program on a hard drive or network system.

INTEGRATING COMPUTER APPLICATIONS INTO YOUR CURRICULUM

The textbook and software can be used either in a classroom environment or on a tutorial basis. Computer availability will principally determine how *Computer Applications* can be best implemented within a particular curriculum. Instructors who have a limited number of computers may elect to cover the theoretical part of the text in class, and then assign computer time to students. Others may find that it is better to restructure the curriculum to include *Computer Applications* when students learn about insurance processing, billing, and collections. When computer labs are available for instruction, the teacher will have the greatest flexibility in determining the course structure.

Schools that do not teach computer skills courses or modules within the medical assisting or medical clerical curriculum can use *Computer Applications* by having the computer science instructors assign the text on a tutorial basis while providing limited instruction. Nevertheless, consideration should be given to eventually integrating the content into the medical assisting or medical clerical curriculum.

A student will need approximately 30 hours of computer time to complete the simulations in the textbook. This does not include Chapter 7, Billing and Collections, and Chapter 8, Insurance Processing.

GETTING STARTED

Software Installation

Before you can run *Patriot Medical® (PM),* the two program disks must be installed on your hard disk. The installation procedure decompresses and copies files from the two program disks onto your hard disk to create the PM program. The two program disks along with documentation for hard drive and network installation are found in back of the Instructor's Guide.

System Requirements

- IBM or compatible PC with at least 4 Mb RAM
- one 5.25-inch or 3.5-inch high density disk drive
- DotMatrix or Laser printer

CHAPTER AIDS

The following section contains a chapter outline, overview, potential problems and suggestions for each chapter in the textbook. The chapter outline and overview provide a brief description of the course content; the troubleshooting sections, *Potential Problems* and *Suggestions* are designed to help you alleviate software problems. You might find it useful to print the latter two sections and discuss them with your students before they begin the activities.

Chapter 1: Developing Computer Competency

CHAPTER OUTLINE
COMPUTERS IN THE MEDICAL OFFICE
COMPUTER-BASED COMMUNICATION SYSTEMS
PERSONAL COMPUTERS
MICROCOMPUTER HARDWARE
     Input Devices
     Processing Devices
     Output Devices
     Storage Devices
OPERATING SYSTEMS
     Disk Operating System
     DOS Versus Windows
ERGONOMIC WORKSTATIONS
PREPARING TO RUN PATRIOT MEDICAL® PROGRAM
     Learning Activity 1–1: Back Up Data Disk
     Learning Activity 1–2: Medical Practice Business Information Folders
COMPUTER SAFETY PROCEDURES
     Backup Files
     Index Files
     Clear Disk Space
REVIEW QUESTIONS

OVERVIEW
This chapter presents basic information about microcomputers. The student learns the names and functions of the major components of a microcomputer. He or she learns how to enter information using the keyboard, producing hard copies from printers, and making backup copies. The computer skills that the student masters in this chapter are needed to complete the simulations in subsequent chapters of the text.

POTENTIAL PROBLEMS
It is important for the student to complete this chapter and the two learning activities included in it in order to be adequately prepared for Chapter 2. The Computer Safety Procedures section, pages 13 to 14 should be stressed. These safety procedures ensure, through the utilities included in the software, that student mistakes and power failure do not result in loss of data. Other problems include not having the printer turned on and on line, disk drive latches not closed, and not having a data disk in the drive.

SUGGESTIONS

For those classes in which students have already completed a number of computer courses, this chapter can be used as a review. The chapter test can be administered to determine their competency. The chapter review questions can be used as a homework assignment and for general discussion.

Chapter 2: Database Entry and Report Printing

CHAPTER OUTLINE

RUNNING THE PATRIOT MEDICAL® PROGRAM
>Learning Activity 2–1: Signing on the PM Program

MASTER FILES
>Charges (CPT Codes)
>>Learning Activity 2–2: CPT Codes
>>Applied Activity 2–1: CPT Codes

>Payments
>>Applied Activity 2–2: Payment Code Master File

>Miscellaneous

>Diagnosis Code (ICD Codes)
>>Learning Activity 2–3: ICD-9 Codes
>>Applied Activity 2–3: ICD-9 Codes

>Referring Providers
>>Learning Activity 2–4: Referring Providers
>>Applied Activity 2–4: Referring Providers

>Providers
>>Applied Activity 2–5: Provider

>Facilities
>>Applied Activity 2–6: Facility

>Insurance
>>Applied Activity 2–7: Insurance

>Modifiers
>>Applied Activity 2–8: Modifiers

>Place of Service
>>Applied Activity 2–9: Place of Service

>Type of Service
>>Applied Activity 2–10: Type of Service

REPORTS
>Learning Activity 2–5: Master File Reports
>Applied Activity 2–11: Master File Reports

REVIEW QUESTIONS

OVERVIEW

The computer skills that the student learned in the previous chapter are needed to complete the activities in the textbook. In this chapter, the student inputs data required for the daily operation of a medical practice. These data include entering the CPT and ICD-9 codes, the name(s) of physician(s) treating the patients as well as other data that are required to automatically generate billing statements, insurance claims, and reports. They also include production of master file reports. Once this information is entered in a medical practice, the files are accessed primarily to view screens, update files, and generate reports.

POTENTIAL PROBLEMS

The student should be careful to follow suggested sign-on procedures and to place his or her data disk in the disk drive. It is also important to select Quit from the Main Menu and completely sign off the program before removing the data disk from the disk drive. Failure to do so, may result in losing data.

Many students have a tendency to complete the activity steps rather rapidly, but they fail to read and understand the explanations in the activities. It is important for the instructor to reinforce the importance of understanding the theoretical concepts of each activity. Accuracy and completeness of data entry followed by verification that all information entered is correct should be stressed as a common practice in a medical setting. These skills should be developed in the classroom setting. The student should understand that data entered are used to generate statements, insurance claims, and to produce various reports. Incomplete or inaccurate information on statements or insurance claims could delay payment to the physician and create unnecessary work for the office staff. The insurance carrier or patient may even refuse to send a check until a corrected claim form is processed. Incorrect or missing CPT and/or ICD-9 codes will cause problems once the daily transactions are entered in subsequent chapters.

SUGGESTIONS

Students should be encouraged to back up their data files at the end of the working day. As an instructor, you may want to produce a disk at the end of each chapter. If a student loses or corrupts their data disk, a copy of your master chapter disk can be used to continue with their computer activities. The importance of placing reports and files in a systematic fashion and in correct folders should also be discussed.

The chapter review questions can be used as a homework assignment and for general discussion. The computer audit is structured to validate the student's computer competency of completeness and accuracy of entered data. The test bank is based on the end-of-chapter review questions in the textbook and computer audits, which in turn are based on the student objectives.

Chapter 3: Patients and Guarantors

CHAPTER OUTLINE
MASTER FILES
  Financial Class
    Applied Activity 3–1: Financial Class
  Billing Cycle
    Applied Activity 3–2: Billing Cycle
  Employers
    Applied Activity 3–3: Employers
  Passwords
  Company
    Applied Activity 3–4: Company
REPORTS
  Applied Activity 3–5: Master Files Reports
  Patients and Guarantors
    Learning Activity 3–1: Patient and Guarantor Files, John Thomas
    Applied Activity 3–6: Patient and Guarantor Files, Debbie G. Conrad
    Applied Activity 3–7: Patient and Guarantor Files, Mary A. Douglas
    Applied Activity 3–8: Patient and Guarantor Files, Carlos N. Giovanni
    Applied Activity 3–9: Patient and Guarantor Files, Tom Kinner
    Applied Activity 3–10: Patient and Guarantor Files, Jack A. Nicklaus
    Applied Activity 3–11: Patient and Guarantor Files, Cathy J. Ramos
REPORTS
  Applied Activity 3–12: Master Files Reports
REVIEW QUESTIONS

OVERVIEW
The purpose of this chapter is to complete the remaining databases in the master files, enter databases for guarantors and patients, print reports for the master files and patient's accounts, and to back up data files.

In the medical office, information that is entered in the patient and guarantor file is obtained from a form that the patient fills out during the initial office visit. These data are used for credit and collections should the account become delinquent. The guarantor entered here will receive the bill and is the responsible party.

POTENTIAL PROBLEMS
Again, some students will have a tendency to complete the activity steps rather rapidly but fail to read and understand the explanations in the activities. It is important for the instructor to continue reinforcing the importance of understanding the theoretical concepts of each activity. Accuracy and completeness of data entry followed by verification that all information entered is correct should be stressed as a common practice in a medical setting. These skills can and should be developed in the classroom setting. Students who do not take adequate time to verify the accuracy of their patient and guarantor entries will experience improper billing reports in subsequent chapters.

The biggest problem some students encounter in this chapter is entering patient and guarantor files correctly. To avoid confusion and frustration, the PM Caution on page 48 should be followed. It is recommended not to begin Learning Activity 3–1, pages 48 to 54 and subsequent patient and guarantor activities unless those activities can be completed in their entirety during a given session. Allow at least 45 minutes to complete Learning Activity 3–1. If a student ends a session in the middle of a patient and guarantor file entry and sign on PM at a later time, the screens and sequence of events will differ slightly. This may cause confusion. Until the student fully understands Figure 3–11 and how to navigate through the various files, it is imperative to follow the PM Caution in this chapter.

SUGGESTIONS

Students must continuously be encouraged to compare their screen entries to the figures in the chapter to verify that data are entered correctly and to read and review the PM Tips Cautions. They should also be encouraged to back up their data files at the end of the working day. As an instructor, you may want to produce a disk at the end of each chapter. If a student loses or corrupts their data disk, a copy of your master chapter disk can be used to continue with their computer activities.

The chapter review questions can be used as a homework assignment and for general discussion. The computer audit is structured to validate student's computer competency of completeness and accuracy of entered data. The test bank is based on the end-of-chapter review questions in the textbook, and computer audits, which in turn are based on the student objectives.

Chapter 4: Insurance and Day Sheet Management

CHAPTER OUTLINE

OVERVIEW

Before the students begin to enter charge and payment transactions on the day sheet, they will verify that the Account Setup and Insurance Template for each patient and guarantor are set up correctly. By doing this, they guarantee that the insurance forms and statements will be sent out correctly in a subsequent chapter. They will also learn to navigate more comfortably through the PM program. This chapter concentrates on posting balance forward transactions, posting a batch payment check, preparing a deposit slip, determining account balances, and reviewing the various options in the Utilities menu.

POTENTIAL PROBLEMS

Even though all patient and guarantor files have been checked to verify accuracy, you might have someone who gets a message on the screen indicating that something is missing from a patient's file. For example, the message "No Insurance Template" lets you know you forgot to create one. If such a message appears on the screen, use the F2 option at the Transaction Entry screen to create a template.

SUGGESTIONS

You may want the students to practice in class, or at their leisure, using the F2 and F4 keys that are discussed in the Navigating Through Posting Session Files on page 83. Great care must be taken not to close the day sheet until it is in balance. Again, students have a tendency to go through this section rather rapidly, close the day sheet, and later find they have errors on the day sheet. All errors on a closed day sheet must be adjusted on the next open day sheet. Depending on the severity of the student's errors, they can also use their backup disk from Chapter 3 to start Chapter 4 again.

The totals and abbreviations on pages 1 and 2 of the day sheet should be discussed. Students should have an understanding of the difference between the month-to-date and year-to-date totals for the practice as well as the patient, insurance, and grand totals. To summarize: The patient totals are the amounts that are directly posted to a patient's accounts, the insurance totals are those amounts that the insurance company has been billed for. The grand total column summarizes the patient and insurance totals.

Students should have a thorough understanding of a batch payment check and the column headings and definitions in Figure 4–22 before they begin Learning Activity 4–5, Day Sheet 2, Posting a Batch Payment Check. This section can be used as a basis for discussion and/or homework. Because of the complexity of Learning Activity 4–5, it is suggested that the student back up their files before beginning this activity and to continue making a backup copy at the end of each learning activity in this chapter. Again, great care should be taken not to rush through the activities.

Day sheet 2 month-to-date, year-to-date, and grand totals should be compared with day sheet 1 so the student can see how the totals transfer from 1 month to the next. If they forget to close a day sheet the month-to-date totals will differ but the grand totals will be the same if they are in balance. They can always go back to close a day sheet.

The chapter review questions can be used as a homework assignment and for general discussion. The computer audit is structured to validate the student's computer competency of completeness and accuracy of entered data. The test bank is based on the end-of-chapter review questions in the textbook, and computer audits, which in turn are based on the student objectives.

The utilities functions are discussed, and even though there are no applicable activities to apply in this section, students can practice the clear disk space and index files functions at this time.

Chapter 5: New Patients and Day Sheet Management

CHAPTER OUTLINE
RECORDING NEW PATIENTS
>   Coordination of Benefits
>> Learning Activity 5–1: Recording Two New Patients with Primary and Secondary
Insurance
>> Medicare Supplemental Insurance
>> Applied Activity 5–1: Recording a Medicare Patient with Supplemental Insurance
>> Applied Activity 5–2: Recording the Patient and Guarantor Files for a New Patient With an
>>>   Established Guarantor

REPORTS
>> Applied Activity 5–3: Master Files Reports

CHARGE AND PAYMENT TRANSACTIONS
>> Learning Activity 5–2: Day Sheet 3, Posting Charge and Payment Transactions and
>>>   Generating Walk-Out Statements
>> Applied Activity 5–4: Continuation of Day Sheet 3
>> Applied Activity 5–5: Print and Balance Day Sheet 3
>> Learning Activity 5–3: Deposit Slip for Day Sheet 3

OVERVIEW
The student continues to gain experience by recording a Medicare patient, patients with primary and secondary insurance, generating reports for patients, posting charges and payments, producing walk-out statements, balancing day sheet 3, and preparing a bank deposit slip.

POTENTIAL PROBLEMS
If a student is unable to print statements, they probably did not configure the statement setup as directed on pages 124 to 125 and as shown in Figure 5–13. Even though the students are guided to be sure their printer is on and on line, sometimes they fail to follow the procedure. Depending on the printer setup, they may experience problems printing their reports. *PM* will allow them to go back after the printer is set up properly to print their walk-out statements.

On the student printouts, the Previous Account Balance section of the Walk-Out Statements for John Thomas, Carlos Giovanni, and Tom Kinner may differ from the figures, but the New Account Balance should be the same. The figures may differ because of the date the transactions were entered. For example, some students may complete the balance forward transactions and payments on one day. Others may complete the balance forward transactions in a given month and complete the payments several months later. Thus, the Previous Account Balance section will differ, but there walk-out statements are still correct if the New Account Balance agrees with the figure.

SUGGESTIONS
Because the Medicare statute designates that a provider of Medicare may not bill a patient until after the provider receives payment from Medicare, students should fully understand the section *Medicare Supplemental Insurance,* page 116 before proceeding with Learning Activity 5–1. The first three activities in this chapter are lengthy. Thus, completing a data file backup after each activity will allow students to use their backups in the event they need to re-enter a learning activity.

Students should review the month-to-date and year-to-date totals for Day Sheet 3 and compare the beginning totals to the ending totals of Day Sheet 2 to see how totals are forwarded and how they accumulate for the year. If they forget to close a day sheet the month-to-date totals will differ but the grand totals will be the same if they are in balance. They can always go back to close a day sheet.

The chapter review questions can be used as a homework assignment and for general discussion. The computer audit is structured to validate the student's computer competency of completeness and accuracy of entered data. The test bank is based on the end-of-chapter review questions in the textbook, and computer audits, which in turn are based on the student objectives.

Chapter 6: Appointment Scheduler

CHAPTER OUTLINE

APPOINTMENT SCHEDULER

REPORTS

Daily/Weekly/Monthly Schedule

REVIEW QUESTIONS

OVERVIEW

This chapter addresses appointment scheduling, which is one of the most important daily functions in a medical office. The student will be taught how to enter appointments, cancel and reschedule appointments, print a daily list of appointments and routing slips, and also about numerous other complexities of the appointment scheduler.

POTENTIAL PROBLEMS

If an error message displays on the monitor while running the Appointment Scheduler, simply follow the instructions on the screen to exit the program. Then complete the steps in Learning Activity 6–2, Indexing scheduling Files, and Learning Activity 6–3, Building Appointment Screens. You may then continue running the Appointment Scheduler.

SUGGESTIONS

Because the Appointment Scheduler is a complex program that processes large amounts of data and uses a great deal of memory (RAM) as its *working space* to hold data and instructions, it is important to sign on PM and go directly to the scheduler. Do not have any other type of program loaded into memory. This is addressed in the "Appointment Scheduler" section, page 138. Students should thoroughly understand this section before proceeding with the learning activities. To avoid error messages, be patient, and do not press any keys while the program is loading or processing data.

To master the appointment scheduler, the student can complete the scheduling of patients in Learning Activities 6–4, pages 142 to 145 and Applied Activity 6–1, pages 145 to 149 on another subsequent month.

Once day sheet 4 is produced, they should review the month-to-date and year-to-date totals and compare the beginning totals to the ending totals of Day Sheet 3. This will fortify their understanding of how totals are forwarded and how they accumulate for the year. If they forget to close a day sheet, the month-to-date totals will differ but the grand totals will be the same. They can always go back to close a day sheet.

The chapter review questions can be used as a homework assignment and for general discussion. The computer audit is structured to validate the student's computer competency of completeness and accuracy of entered data. The test bank is based on the end-of-chapter review questions in the textbook, and computer audits, which in turn are based on the student objectives.

Chapter 7: Billing and Collections

CHAPTER OUTLINE
COMPARISON OF A COMPUTERIZED AND A NONCOMPUTERIZED BILLING SYSTEM
MAINTAINING ACCURATE RECORDS
THE PEGBOARD SYSTEM
BILLING
    Statement Preparation
    Billing Schedule
ACCOUNT AGING
COLLECTION PROCESSES THAT ORIGINATE IN THE OFFICE
    Written Billing and Collections Policies
    Collection Notices
    Telephone Collections
SPECIAL PROBLEMS
    Skips
    Bankruptcies
    Write-Offs
    Claims Against Estates
COLLECTION PROCESSES THAT ORIGINATE OUTSIDE THE OFFICE
    Collection Resources
    Using Collection Agencies
    Using the Courts
ETHICAL AND LEGAL IMPLICATIONS OF THE COLLECTION PROCESS
    Truth in Lending Act (Regulation Z of the Consumer Protection Act of 1969)
    Fair Credit Reporting Act of 1971
    Equal Credit Opportunity Act of 1975
    Notice on Use of Telephone for Debt Collecting (Federal Communications Commission)
PATIENT TEACHING CONSIDERATION
REVIEW QUESTIONS

OVERVIEW
The purpose of this chapter is to develop the students' ability to accept responsibility for the billing and collection systems in the physician's office and to help them establish skills for such activities in addition to pointing out the importance of managing financial matters. Various collection procedures are covered as well as the legal implications of the collections process.

POTENTIAL PROBLEMS AND SUGGESTIONS
There are no computer activities in this chapter so the computer program is not used. In previous chapters data have been entered into the computer to maintain a billing and collection system. For the student to establish the required skill and to realize the importance of managing financial matters, various aspects of the billing and collection process have been brought out in this chapter. The student will produce applicable collections reports in other chapters, i.e., the aging report in Chapter 9.

The chapter review questions can be used as a homework assignment and for general discussion. The test bank is based on the end-of-chapter review questions in the textbook, which in turn are based on the student objectives.

Chapter 8: Insurance Processing

CHAPTER OUTLINE

CODING SYSTEMS
> ICD-9 Coding
> CPT Coding
> The CPT Manual

PROCESSING A HEALTH INSURANCE CLAIM FORM
> Special Company Insurance Forms
> Optical Scanning
> Super Bills

GOVERNMENT-SPONSORED INSURANCE PROGRAMS
> Medicare
> > *Eligibility*
> > *Processing Claims for Medicare*
> > *Calculations and Rationale Recap*
> Learning Activity 8–1: Medicare Claim Form
> Medicaid
> > *Processing Claims for Medicaid*
> Medicare-Medicaid
> Champus and Champva
> Workers' Compensation
> > *Processing Workers' Compensation Reports*

GROUP-SPONSORED OR INDIVIDUAL PLANS

MANAGED CARE
> Health Maintenance Organizations
> Individual Practice Associations or Individual Professional Plans
> Preferred Provider Organizations
> Blue Cross and Blue Shield Programs
> Major Medical Plans

SECONDARY INSURANCE BILLING

CLAIM REJECTION

WRITE-OFFS

REVIEW QUESTIONS

OVERVIEW

This chapter covers ICD-9 and CPT coding systems and major types of health insurance programs. The government-sponsored insurance programs, Medicare, Medicaid, Champus and Champva, Workers' Compensation are included in this chapter as well as Managed Care Plans, HMOs, IPAs, IPPs, PPOs, Blue Cross and Blue Shield Programs, major medical plans, and secondary insurance billing.

POTENTIAL PROBLEMS AND SUGGESTIONS

There are no computer activities provided for this chapter. Some of the problems and suggestions for filing insurance claims are covered in the Claim Rejection section on pages 209 to 210. These should be reviewed with the students. In Learning Activity 8–1, the student has the opportunity to manually complete a HCFA 1500 claim form. The chapter review questions can be used as a homework assignment and for general discussion. The test bank is based on the end-of-chapter review questions in the textbook, which in turn are based on the student objectives.

Chapter 9: Billing and Practice Management

OUTLINE

OVERVIEW

The purpose of this chapter is to generate bills and statements sent to guarantors and their insurance companies to produce reports that supply the practice with financial information. Students are also exposed to posting a batch payment check, balancing the day sheet, and bank deposit slips.

POTENTIAL PROBLEMS

Unless the data entered in previous activities were verified as accurate, the reports, statements, and insurance claims will not be correct. This can be avoided if the student follows instructions in the prior activities and verifies data entries within each chapter.

In Learning Activity 9–3: Statements, page 215, the dunning messages on the student's hard copies may differ from the answer key in appendix D depending on the dates the transactions were entered.

In Learning Activity 9–10: Aging Accounts and Printing an Aged Accounts Receivable Report, page 228, students who do not change the system date as directed will find that their hard copies do not show a 60-day distribution as illustrated in Figure 9–12. Also, the 30-, 60-, 90-, and 120-day distribution columns will differ according to the date the transactions were entered. However, the total columns and accounts receivable listed on page 2 should be the same as Figure 9–12.

Unless the student closes the month as directed in Learning Activity 9–11, Closing the Month, on page 230, their day sheet month to date totals as shown in Figure 9–15 will differ. However, their year-to-date totals should match Figure 9–15.

If "All Charges on Insurance Form Number 5 have Insurance Payments Applied to them," displays on the student's in Applied Activity 9–2: Posting an Insurance Payment from Blue Cross, Item 20–23, page 233, select the option Return Without Deleting. This statement may display because Tom Kinner has a -96.00 patient balance. The student probably did not follow the instructions in item 33 to "Transfer This Item to Patient Balance."

SUGGESTIONS

Incorrect data that show on the reports, statements, and insurance claims can be corrected. The student should edit incorrect entries and reprint the appropriate report, statement, or insurance claim. Editing guides are found in the chapter that data are originally entered. Activities throughout the textbook provide numerous figures and illustrations to compare data entry as well as editing procedures to make corrections that can also be used to make corrections.

A HCFA 1500 transparency can be produced by using the standard HCFA 1500 form. Students can overlay the transparency on the insurance claim(s) that were generated to see how the data align in the proper boxes. Do not use the HCFA 1500 form since it has been sized down and will not overlay properly on the printed claims. Pre-printed HCFA 1500 forms can be purchased from a local supply store and used to demonstrate the printing of claims in a medical practice.

ANSWERS TO REVIEW QUESTIONS

Each textbook chapter contains review questions. These questions are answered thoroughly in this section. The answers provide the instructor with instant feedback to check the understanding of concepts in each chapter. The reviews are intended to be used for either class work or homework for your students. They also serve as the basis for the chapter tests

Chapter 1: Developing Computer Competency

1. Name the three main categories of computers and describe each.

   Microcomputers are the smallest, least powerful, and least expensive computers. They are also known as personal computers. Minicomputers are quicker in processing and are designed for small and mid-size businesses. Mainframes are the largest, fastest, and most expensive computers with powerful memory capacity. They are used by large corporations or medical facilities.

2. What are two common forms of output devices on microcomputers? Also, give an example of output in the medical office.

   Two common forms of output devices are printers and monitors. Examples of output in a physician's office are insurance forms and statements

3. Describe the differences between a hard drive, floppy disk drive, and CD-ROM drive.

   Each is a type of storage device on a microcomputer; the floppy disk is small, inexpensive, and portable. The hard disk drive is built in to the computer and cannot be removed; however, it holds more data and is more expensive than a floppy disk. The CD-ROM drive has a greater capacity for storage than floppy disks and is portable, but information cannot be added to a CD-ROM drive on a personal computer.

4. List five safety precautions when handling a diskette.

   - *Don't touch the disk surface that reads information*
   - *Don't use near a magnetic field*
   - *Use only a felt tip pen to write on the disk*
   - *Don't expose the disk to hot or cold temperatures*
   - *Don't put heavy objects on the disk*
   - *Store disks in protective covers*

5. Why is it necessary to produce backup disks daily?

   Floppy disks have a limited lifetime and eventually wear out. Technical difficulties and power failures also cause data to be lost. You may lose your Master Disk or it may become damaged or corrupted. In a medical office backup disks are frequently stored either in a fireproof safe or taken off the premises.

6. Name five uses of computers in the medical field.

> *Patient billing, appointment scheduling, diagnose illnesses, monitor vital signs, process patient medical records, producing and storing statistical data to monitor epidemics.*

7. Explain how E-mail (electronic mail) operates and give an illustration of its use in the medical office.

> *A message is sent by computer to another computer via a modem, a device used in telecommunication. A medical office may file insurance claims and correspond with other businesses via E-mail.*

8. What are the four basic functions of microcomputer hardware components?

> *input, processing, output, and storage*

9. Describe the following keys on the keyboard: NumLock, arrow keys, Print Screen, and function keys.

> *The NumLock key activates the numbers on the numeric keypad. The four arrow keys allow the cursor to move one space or row in the direction of the arrow. The Print Screen key allows the contents of the screen to be printed. The Function keys are used for specific tasks in a program.*

10. Explain the purpose of these two safety features: index files and clear disk space.

> *Indexing files will allow files that have been corrupted to be put back in order. Clearing disk space will physically remove deleted information from a storage device (hard drive, network, or floppy), thus making room for more data and index files. The Clear Disk Space function also indexes the files.*

11. Which type of printer can print more pages per minute, dot matrix or laser?

> *Laser*

12. Why would a medical office choose to file insurance forms electronically?

> *It is faster and the turnaround time is quicker. Paperwork is reduced. Soon the federal government will require Medicare and Medicaid be filed electronically.*

13. Designate whether each of the following is an input component, processing component, or output component:

      a)   **Keyboard** — *input*
      b)   **Printer** — *output*
      c)   **Monitor** — *output*
      d)   **CPU** — *processing*
      e)   **Disk drive** — *input and output*

Chapter 2: Database Entry and Report Writing

1. What key(s) is used to scroll through the main menus on the PM program?

   arrow keys

2. In order to add data to any of the files, which command must be entered from the menu bar at the bottom of the screen?

   A/Add

3. What key is able to take you to the end of a file?

   PgDn

4. *(a)* How many digits are there in a CPT code? *(b)* What are CPT codes used for?

   a) *They are five-digit numbers that correspond to terms describing medical services provided and procedures performed by physicians.*

   b) *Besides describing medical services, they give the charges for each procedure.*

5. To sign off the PM program, what steps must be followed? What could happen if the program is not exited properly?

   Return to the Main Menu, scroll to and select Quit. Then press Enter. Then remove the data disk after completely signing off. Files could be corrupted or lost if the program is not signed off properly.

6. Describe these screens: a) Drive Selection screen; b) Welcome screen; c) PM Program Information screen; d) Main Menu opening screen.

   a) *The **Drive Selection Screen** allows the user to enter the letter of the drive that holds the data disk.*

   b) *The **Welcome Screen** is where the user must enter the correct password to access the PM program.*

   c) *The **PM Program Information screen** contains the name of the software company, the version number of the software, and copyright warnings.*

   d) *The **Main Menu opening screen** displays the six main menu choices and the Daily Entry pull down menu.*

7. Describe these five parts of a screen: (a) Main Menu, (b) pull-down menu, (c) pop-up menu, (d) hot key, and (e) menu bar at bottom of screen.

    a)   *The **Main Menu** displays six menu selections that provide access to all of PM's programs and correspond with six routine office activities.*

    b)   *A **pull-down menu** is a list of commands that "drops down" from a menu bar at the top of the screen.*

    c)   *A **pop-up menu** appears when more selections from the pull down menu are available.*

    d)   *A **hot key** is a key that is used to access or activate a program.*

    e)   *The **menu bar** at the bottom of the screen gives choices such as F/find, V/view, E/edit, A/add, D/delete, and R/return.*

8. What happens after you press **R** for Return from the bottom menu bar?

    You are returned to the previous screen.

9. If no information needs to be entered in a field, how do you advance to the next field?

    Press Enter

10. Which command on the menu bar at the bottom of the screen allows you to make changes in a file?

    E/Edit

11. What is the procedure to save a file?

    Press PgDn and press Enter

12. What is the purpose of each file listed below:

    a)   *The **Payment Code Master File** stores payment codes that are used for billing.*

    b)   *The **Diagnosis Code Master File** stores all the medical diagnoses commonly used by the medical practice.*

    c)   *The **Provider Master File** maintains information needed to produce insurance forms and statements for each provider of service (physician) in the practice.*

    d)   *The **Insurance Master File** stores data files of all the insurance companies billed by the practice.*

    e)   *The **Type of Service (TOS) Code Master File** stores the codes for the types of services performed, such as medical and surgical services.*

13. If you had a question concerning one of the fields on a screen, where would you find information explaining the fields?

> *Read the explanation of the field at the bottom of the screen when the cursor is positioned on the field; refer to PM Documentation that is provided to your instructor.*

14. (a) Which Main Menu option generates reports? (b) List and briefly describe four printing formats. (c) What is the preview option?

> *a)* *All reports are generated from the Reports option of the Main Menu.*
>
> *b)* *The four printing formats are detailed (with complete information), condensed (with brief summary of information), totals only (lists totals only), and mailing labels (prints on mailing labels).*
>
> *c)* *The preview option allows the user to view the report on the screen before sending it to the printer.*

15. Tell how information from printed reports can be valuable in a medical practice.

> *The information from reports provides demographic information and also helps determine the financial health of the practice.*

16. Where are CPT and Accounting Codes used to complete the billing process stored in PM?

> *Charge Code Master File*

17. Which Master File stores batch entry and zip codes used most frequently by your patients?

> *Miscellaneous*

18. Where is information on all sources of referrals to your medical practice stored?

> *Master Referring Provider File*

19. How many Modifier Codes are stored in your Modifier Master File? Describe each one briefly.

> *There are three: -22 (Required more time than usual); -81 (Required minimal services of an assistant surgeon); and -90 (Laboratory procedure performed by an outside lab).*

20. What is the difference between the Facility Master File and the Place of Service Code Master File?

> *The Place of Service Code Master File stores information about all medical facilities where the physician treats or consults with patients, including*

his/her main office. The Facility Master File stores information on all the outside facilities that the physician sends patients to for services, i.e., a Medical Laboratory so patient can have a battery of lab tests.

Chapter 3: Patients and Guarantors

1. What type of information is entered in the Billing Cycle Master File?

    A code number is entered with a description of the code. These codes designate how often the billing will be performed.

2. Why is it necessary to keep a file of all the employers your patients may work for?

    Reports can be generated by employer groups.

3. What are the two purposes of the Password Master File?

    It is used to identify anyone who enters data into PM and to restrict users to certain areas of PM.

4. Where will the information from the company file automatically print?

    On statements, invoices, insurance forms, and report headings.

5. The Reports Menu generates reports on all the data. Why is this an important feature?

    This allows better management of the medical practice and provides a visual to verify accuracy of data input.

6. Will the guarantor number on your screen match those in the figures and databases? Why or why not?

    Numbers may differ depending on the sequence patients were entered, whether a file was deleted, etc.

7. If you interrupt the printing of reports, what error message could display on your monitor? What procedure would correct this?

    *Error USING **xxxx.dbf**, Clear Disk Space would correct it.*

8. What would the following error message indicate: "Not ready reading Drive A or B -- Abort, Retry, Fail?"

    The data disk is not placed in the proper drive.

9. Once all of the Master Files are set up, what is the next step in computerizing a medical office?

    Patients with a balance forward must be entered in the system.

10. If you did not know the insurance company code of a new guarantor, how would you locate it from the Add New Guarantor screen?

    Enter a "?" in the insurance company field, which will access the Master File. Select the proper code and return to the Add New Guarantor Screen.

11. What is the difference between a patient and a guarantor? Are all guarantors patients?

    A patient is the person who receives medical treatment; a guarantor is the person who guarantees to pay for all charges on an account. A patient can be a guarantor, but not all guarantors are patients.

12. What option of the PM program saves you from retyping the same data from the New Guarantor File to the New Patient File?

    CARRY INFORMATION option.

13. How is a patient's account number determined in PM?

    The first three letters from the last name and the first three letters from the first name make up the account number.

14. List the general steps in adding a new guarantor (who is also a new patient) with a balance forward.

    - *Access and complete the Add New Guarantor Screen.*
    - *Use CARRY INFORMATION to New Patient option.*
    - *Complete New Patient screen.*
    - *Verify the account set up.*
    - *Create an insurance template.*

15. What function key is used to access Patient options and Insurance Template from the Patient Search file and where is the command located on the screen?

    The F2 key; it is found at the bottom of the Patient Search screen.

Chapter 4: Insurance and Day Sheet Management

1. What is the purpose of open-time accounting?

    Open-item accounting provides flexibility of posting payments to specific charges. This gives you line-by-line detail of all transactions.

2. Which of the Main Menu items and options are accessed to enter balance-forward transactions?

    The Daily Entry menu and the Post Transactions option.

3. What is the value of the "?" feature in the PM program?

    The "?" feature will display codes and descriptions stored in the file and allow you to quickly return to the working screen.

4. What option on the Daily Entry menu is accessed to edit transactions on a day sheet?

    Updating Transactions

5. After closing several day sheets, how do you know which day sheet is the open or active one?

    The open day sheet appears last on the Daily Balancing Sheet.

6. How do you make corrections to a closed day sheet?

    Corrections must be entered on a subsequent open day sheet.

7. How is an insured patient informed of the amount of coverage paid to your office by his or her insurance company?

    The insurance carrier sends an EOB (explanation of benefits) indicating what portion of the charge is reimbursed and what portion is the patient's responsibility.

8. What housekeeping tasks are usually completed monthly with medical billing software?

    Index files, Clear Disk Space, Apply Finance Charges, Balance Update

9. What option from the Utilities menu should be used if there is a power failure or if you have problems locating data?

    Index Files or Clear Disk Space

10. What is the purpose of the Clear Disk Space option on the Utilities menu?

Clear Disk Space permanently removes data from a storage device (hard drive, floppy, or network), thus making room for more data and index files.

Chapter 5: New Patients and Day Sheet Management

1. What does COB mean?

    Coordination of Benefits is a clause found in insurance policies, which requires that insurers coordinate the payment of services if a patient is covered by two or more medical insurance policies.

2. What is the difference between the designation of primary and secondary carrier?

    The primary carrier is billed first, and any charges remaining will be billed to the secondary carrier.

3. When entering new patients with a guarantor that is already established as a patient, you are instructed to select the Do Not Carry Information option. Why are you instructed to do so?

    The guarantor is not the same person as the patient.

4. What key item on the Patient Account Setup for Medicare allows for bills to be sent after Medicare has paid their share?

    The billing mode is I, not A.

5. When Medicare patients have supplemental insurance, who is considered the primary carrier?

    If a person is older than 65 years of age and retired, Medicare is the primary carrier. If the patient is 65 to 69 years of age and still working, then Medicare is secondary to the employer's group plan.

6. What menu and option is accessed to enter payments and charges?

    Daily Entry menu. Then select, Post Transactions option.

7. What menu and options allow you to produce a hard copy of a day sheet and a deposit slip?

    The Daily Entry menu. Then select either Daily Deposit Slip or the Day Sheet option.

8. What occurs when a day sheet is closed?

    MTD and YTD totals print, and transactions that may be incorrect will need to be corrected on a subsequent day sheet.

9. What two options can you select to enter patient data?

    *The **Patients** option from the Master Files menu, and the **Add Patients** option from the Daily Entry menu.*

10. Why should patient data be entered accurately into the computer?

Lack of information or incomplete information could cause rejection from the insurance carriers, which results in delayed payment.

11. Can you finish the Insurance Template before completing the guarantor and/or patient files?

No, because no guarantor/patient data exists in PM until those files are completed.

12. What figure in Chapter 3 is useful to determine the sequential steps to enter a new patient and guarantor?

Figure 3–11, Summary of the process for entering a new patient and guarantor.

13. List the sequential steps to enter data for a new patient.

Select Add New Patient; complete New Guarantor/New Patient files; complete Account Setup and Insurance Template

14. What figure in Chapter 3 is useful to determine how to complete a patient/guarantors file if you entered the guarantor on one day and go back to complete the file the next day?

Figure 3–11, Summary of the process for entering a new patient and guarantor.

15. Will your Guarantor# fields match the ones in the figures and databases? If no, why not?

PM automatically assigns guarantors numbers in sequential order. If you did not enter a guarantors in the exact order listed in the activity or if you deleted a guarantor, your sequence and assigned number will be different. Do not be concerned if your numbers differ.

Chapter 6: Appointment Scheduler

1. What is the advantage of having an appointment scheduling system?

   A smooth flow of patient traffic is required for an efficient medical office.

2. In what two locations can you access the appointment scheduler?

   *From the **Daily Entry Menu** and the **Post Transactions** option.*

3. Explain how the arrow keys help to navigate the scheduler.

   The right arrow moves one day to the right and the left arrow moves one day to the left. The up arrow moves to the day above on the calendar and the down arrow moves one day below.

4. What will the PgDn command perform in the Scheduler?

   It will allow you to access prior months.

5. What will occur if you book an appointment in a prior month, and why?

   The appointment scheduler will not permit you to book an appointment in a prior month. An error message might result if you try to do so.

6. How will the <Note> option in the scheduler be useful?

   It permits you to list a special reminder on a specific day of the calendar.

7. List four different types of appointments stored in the PM system.

   New Patient, Established Patient, Flu Vaccine, Postoperative Care, etc.

8. When there is no Type code for an appointment, what should you do?

   *Select the code **OTHERS**, and at the **Comment:** field type the specific description for the visit.*

9. Can new patients be scheduled if they are not recorded in the PM system? If yes, specify how.

   Yes, *patients can be scheduled, but the option "Add Patient Later" must be selected and the type code should be **NEWPAT**.*

10. What is the difference between editing a 15-minute appointment and a 30-minute appointment?

    *Once the appointment is highlighted, for the 30-minute appointment, **D** (for Details) is selected to edit. For the 15-minute appointment, **Add Appointment** is selected.*

11. What report is generated most frequently from the Scheduler and what are the ranges available to print?

   The Daily/Weekly/Monthly Schedule is run most often. It can generate lists for one day or a range of days. It can list a specific type of appointment and can list in detail or summary. This report also lists the new patients.

12. What is the purpose of the routing slip and when should it be printed?

   The Route Slip provides a list of all services performed during an office visit, including CPT codes and Diagnoses codes. It should be printed prior to the office visit and clipped to the patient's chart.

13. How would you display the Transaction Detail screen for Debbie Conrad?

   *At the Daily Entry Menu or at the Transaction Entry screen, select **Update Transactions**. Then enter **CONDEB** at the patient account number field to display the Transaction Detail screen, then press F4 (command at the bottom of the screen).*

14. When the Transaction Detail screen is displayed, what command would you select to display her current balance?

   F4/ACCOUNT SUMMARY. This is displayed at the bottom of the Transaction Detail screen.

15. Once you have completed all the activities in this chapter, list CONDEB's current balance.

   Her current balance is $695. This can be obtained in two ways: From the Master Files menu, Patients option, or from the Daily Entry menu, Update Transactions option.

   Master Files menu: Select Patients, V to view account. The Total Due: shows 695.00

   Daily Entry menu: Select Update Transactions, The unpaid balances show 15, 35, 645, which equals 695.00. Now press F4 Account Summary. The Unpaid Insurance amount shows 695.00

Chapter 7: Billing and Collections

1. Define the following terms:

   a) **Cash flow**—*checks or cash received by the practice*

   b) **One-write system**—*pegboard accounting system consisting of a flat writing surface with a series of evenly spaced pegs along its left edge. This system generates all the financial records needed for each transaction with a single entry transferred onto the various other forms through use of a pressure-sensitive noncarbon paper.*

   c) **Aging schedule**—*a record of all patient account balances, when the charges originated, the most recent payment, and any special notes concerning the account.*

   d) **Straight bankruptcy**—*a type of bankruptcy under the direct protection of the court in which all collection procedures must cease.*

   e) **Wage earner's bankruptcy**—*a patient who files for wage earner's bankruptcy agrees to pay a fixed amount to the bankruptcy referee, from who all creditors than receive distributions. Creditors may not garner wages or in any way proceed against the debtor who is under a wage earner's plan.*

   f) **Garnishment**—*withholding of a specified amount from an employee's wages to satisfy a debt.*

   g) **Litigation**—*a lawsuit.*

   h) **Bilateral agreement**—*an agreement between two parties; outlines legal obligations of both.*

   i) **Skips**—*a debtor who moves and leaves no forwarding address.*

2. How can the office staff inform patients tactfully of office payment policies?

   - *Small sign in conspicuous area of office stating, "All services should be paid for in full at the time of service unless other arrangements have been made in advance."*

   - *Give patient pre-addressed mailing envelope in which to return payment and explain payment policy.*

   - *Additional answers may vary: Inform patient at time appointment is scheduled of payment policy; office may include payment and insurance collection policies section in patient information brochure.*

3. What documents are simultaneously generated with the "one-write" accounting system?

   For patient accounts: *Daily earnings summary, deposit slip, ledger card, and patient charge and receipt slip.*

For payments: *cash payment journal, a voucher, a check, voucher proof of expenditures, and disbursements categorizes cash expenditures.*

4. When is the best time to collect fees from patients?

    At the time service is rendered. This improves cash flow; statistically, the longer a debt is owed the lesser the probability of collection.

5. Explain the cyclic billing method.

    A method of billing in which a portion of the statements are mailed out at various times during the month. Eliminates the burden of preparing and mailing all statements on a single day and evens cash flow over entire month.

6. What valuable information is provided by an analysis of the aging schedule?

    Trends in length of time, outstanding amounts collected, and insurance claims outstanding emerge. This information also allows determination of collection percentage for specified time period.

7. Name some important considerations in selecting a collection agency.

    Investigate the agency's collection practices and reliability. Further, consider the agency's philosophy and operational methods. Additionally, request references and contact other physicians who utilize this particular agency. Finally, other considerations are the ethics, promptness, and efficiency of the agency. Resources for evaluation of these considerations may be the local Better Business Bureau and state and national organizations or credit agencies.

8. Once an account is referred to a collection agency, should the physician's office continue to send the patient statements?

    No.

9. Name six items of information that must be contained in the written agreement for Regulation Z.

    - *Total amount of the debt*
    - *The amount of the down payment*
    - *The date each payment is due*
    - *The amount of each payment and any finance charges. Finance charges must be expressed as an annual percentage rate.*
    - *The date of the final payment.*

10. Name some helpful do's and don'ts for telephone collection

> **DO:**
> *Call the patient during reasonable hours.*
> *Make certain you are talking to the correct person before you identify yourself and the nature of the call.*
> *Keep a positive and friendly attitude.*
> *Be courteous and firm when asking for payment.*
> *Get a specific commitment from the patient as to the amount that will be paid and the date it will be received. State "I have made a note that we will have a check from you in the amount of _____ by April 20."*
> *Provide the patient with the name and address of the physician.*
> *Notify the physician immediately if there is any patient dissatisfaction so that steps may be taken to alleviate potential litigation.*
>
> **DO NOT:**
> *Discuss the nature of the call with anyone but the debtor.*
> *Make threats.*

11. Explain the Equal Credit Opportunity Act of 1975.

> *Federal legislation prohibiting discrimination in the granting of credit. Credit must be extended solely on the ability to pay. A patient's race, religion, and economic status cannot be used a criteria to deny credit.*

12. What information should be included in patient teaching regarding office payment-for-service policies?

> *Patient should be informed of the following:*
> *How to make payment (e.g., check, cash, or credit card)*
> *The consequences of late payment or nonpayment*

Chapter 8: Insurance Processing

1. Define the following terms:

    a) *Reimbursement*—*payment for services rendered, sent either to the patient or to the provider of service.*

    b) *ICD-9-CM*—*International Classification of Diseases, Adapted Revision 9, Clinical Modification; usually shortened to ICD. The code number assigned to a specific disease or disease complex.*

    c) *Diagnosis*—*description of the patient's medical problem. Based on physician's assessment of information acquired while taking the patient history and from the physical examination.*

    d) *Current Procedural Terminology (CPT)*—*a listing of descriptive terms and numeric identifying codes and modifiers used for reporting medical services and procedures performed by physicians or other providers of medical services.*

    e) *Beneficiary*—*a person designated to receive a specified cash payment upon the policyholder's accidental or natural death.*

    f) *Participating providers*—*provider of medical care who has entered into a contract with an organization, the government, or an insurance company to provide medical care to enrolled subscribers. The provider agrees to accept the insurance company's approved fee for each medical service.*

    g) *Assignment of insurance benefits*—*authorization by policy holder or patient to allow the insurance company to pay claim benefits directly to the provider of care.*

    h) *Deductible*—*amount of covered expenses a policy holder must incur each year before the insurance company is obligated to pay benefits.*

    i) *Copayment*—*insurance program provision requiring the sharing of medical costs with the policy holder. A small flat rate may be payable when services are rendered (e.g., $3–$5), or a percentage of the total benefits (e.g., patient pays 20% of costs and insurance reimburses 80%).*

    j) *Allowable charges*—*maximum amount reimbursed by insurance carrier for each procedure or service provided.*

    k) *Primary carrier*—*the insurance carrier that is billed first when a patient or responsible party (RP), also known as a guarantor, holds multiple insurance policies.*

2. What is a reciprocity program?

    An arrangement between two or more insurance programs in different states whereby the program in one state will accept an insurance claim from the program in another state for payment.

3. What does *explanation of benefits (EOB)* mean?

    It is an attachment to the insurance payment check explaining what benefits were paid or why portions of the bill were excluded from payment.

4. What are the names of the three major federal government healthcare programs?

    Medicare, Medicaid, Workers' Compensation, and CHAMPUS

5. Who are the patients served by the Medicare program?

    Patients who are 65 years and older and are eligible for social security; patients who have been disabled for 2 or more years; blind patients; patients with end-stage renal disease.

6. Mrs. Komma has Medicare coverage Parts A and B. Treatment by her physician, Dr. Kenner, included an abdominal hysterectomy with an incidental appendectomy. Dr. Kenner's actual charge was $1250.00. Medicare allowed an amount of $1150.00. Mrs. Komma has not met her deductible for the current year. Dr. Kenner has agreed to accept assignment for this claim.

    a) **What is the write-off amount?**

Actual Charge	*$1250.00*
Medicare Allowed Amount	*-1150.00*
Write-off amount	*$100.00*

    b) **What is the expected payment from Medicare?**

Medicare Allowed Amount:	*$1150.00*
Minus Unmet Deductible	*-100.00*
Amount Considered for payment by Medicare	*$1050.00*
Multiplied by 80%	*x .80*
Expected Medicare Payment	*$840.00*

    c) **What is the expected payment from Mrs. Komma?**

Medicare's allowed amount:	*$1150.00*
Minus unmet deductible	*-100.00*
Amount considered for payment by Medicare	*$1050.00*

Unmet deductible	*+$100.00*
Expected payment from	*$310.00*
Mrs. Komma	

VERIFY YOUR ANSWER

Write-off Amount
Expected Payment from Medicare
Expected Payment from Patient
Equals Amount of Actual Charge

EXPLANATION OF ANSWER

Write-off amount:

Actual Charge	*$1250.00*
Medicare Allowed Amount	*-1150.00*
Write-off amt =	*$100.00*

EXPECTED PAYMENT FROM MEDICARE

Medicare Allowed Amount	*$1150.00*
Minus Unmet Deductible	*- 100.00*
Amount considered for	*$1050.00*
for Medicare reimbursement	
Multiplied by 80%	*x .80*
Equals Expected Medicare	*$840.00*
Payment	

EXPECTED PAYMENT FROM PATIENT

Medicare Allowed Amount	*$1150.00*
Minus Unmet Deductible	*-100.00*
Equals	*$1050.00*
Multiplied by 20%	*x.20*
Equals	*$210.00*
Plus unmet deductible	*+$100.00*
Equals Expected Payment	
From Patient	*$310.00*

Chapter 9: Billing and Practice Management

1. Why were statements printed for all accounts except those of Helen Gunn and David Michaels?

   *Helen Gunn is a Medicare patient. Her account setup designates an **I** for the billing mode as required by Medicare. Therefore, she will not receive a bill until Medicare reimburses the practice for her charges.*

   David Michaels is not a patient and does not have transactions posted on his account. Therefore, the program does not generate a statement for him. However, the statement for his dependent, Lisa Michaels, is generated and it is sent to David Michaels since he is the guarantor.

2. What commands would you enter to view an individual statement?

   *Select **V** for view and **M** for more to view the entire statement.*

3. What two fields must show a Y in order for insurance forms to print?

   *The **As:** and **Ins:** field must show a **Y**. Refer to Figure 9–5 on page 219.*

4. When the Insurance Transaction Holding File displays this message, "There are not records in the Insurance Holding File," what does it indicate?

   This message alerts you that the insurance forms are now ready for processing.

5. What is the purpose of the Scan Forms option?

   The Scan Forms option provides a list of all pending insurance forms on file that have not been fully paid.

6. If you need to reprint a batch of insurance forms, how do you change the status?

   Complete the following steps:
   - *From the Insurance Menu, press **S** to select Scan Forms.*
   - *Highlight the account number, then press **E** to Edit.*
   - *From the Insurance Form# screen, scroll to Print, and press Enter.*
   - *From the Insurance Form Print pop-up menu, press Enter to select Change Print Status.*
   - *At the highlighted Not Prntd option, press Enter to engage the Not Prntd status.*
   - *When you are finished, press the hot key **R** for return.*

7. Which two options in the Insurance Menu permit you to create an individual insurance form?

> *From the Insurance menu select the following options:*
> *Manual Form Entry or Print Forms, ( ) Single Patient Form*

8. Give three advantages of electronic claims transmissions.

> *Claims are processed quickly, in a matter of hours; claims are paid faster; eliminates*
> *tremendous amount of paper work; requires fewer billing clerks; cost of postage,*
> *insurance, follow-up correspondence, etc., is greatly reduced.*

9. What is the difference between the carrier-direct system and the clearinghouse system?

> *Carrier direct system: Offices that have their own computer system lease a terminal*
> *from the insurance carrier. Claims are then processed directly via modem.*

> *Clearinghouse system: Also, referred to as a third-party administrator (TPA)*
> *redistributes the processed claims to various insurance carriers, including*
> *government-sponsored insurance programs. The clearinghouse usually checks to*
> *verify that each claim contains the information required by the carrier to which the*
> *claim is going.*

10. Does the office staff need to be present when electronic claims are transmitted with PM?

> *No, the office staff does not have to be present. The office staff may preset a time*
> *tied to your computer clock to automatically call your payer to transmit claims*
> *without your staff's presence or at an off-peak time.*

11. What is the function of the Productivity/Analysis Report option?

> *It summarizes the volume of procedures performed in a medical practice, listing to*
> *whom and when these procedures were performed. This report is run at the end of*
> *each month after the last day sheet of the month has been closed.*

12. Give an example of how a Productivity/Analysis Report can provide specific information about a medical practice.

> *These reports are designed to isolate groups of patients and procedures that were*
> *performed on them. Statistical data can be used from these reports for medical*
> *research, for determining geographical distribution of prevalent diseases, and for*
> *predicting epidemics.*

13. What key pieces of information are included on an aging schedule?

> *Lists patients' account balances, when the charges originated, the most recent*
> *payment date, and any special notes concerning the account. These data are*
> *obtained from the patient accounts and are automatically sorted by PM into 30-, 60-,*
> *90-, and 120-day periods. All of this information is used to prepare an aging*
> *schedule each month.*

14. How do you change the system date in PM?

> *Utilities menu; System Date*

15. Explain what the system date is.

> *The system date is the current date to which your computer defaults.*

COMPUTER AUDITS

Specially designed computer audits are structured to validate a student's computer competency at the end of chapters 2, 3, 4, 5, 6, and 9. These audits with answer keys make it easy to determine if the student is ready to progress to a subsequent chapter and to validate if they have completed the chapter.

Chapter 2: Database Entry and Report Writing

The following is a mock or practice audit. This can be administered to students so that they will become familiar with subsequent computer audits that are assessed for grading purposes.

Suggested Time Limit: 15 to 20 minutes

1. How many codes do you have in the Charge Code Master File?

    19 (15 CPT codes; 4 accounting codes)

2. List the POS code for 42821, Tonsil & Adenoidectomy.

    2

3. List the User Code and CPT code for Sigmoidoscopy, Flexible, Diagnostic?

    User Code: SIGMOI; CPT code: 45330

4. List the Type fields for the accounting codes, and copy the explanation of this field by displaying an accounting code on your screen.

    Type field: IW; Explanation of Type field: Type of Charge: PW (Patient W/O); IW (Insurance W/O); or Leave Blank.

    The explanation is listed at the bottom of your screen when the cursor is positioned at the Type field.

5. What is the payment code for a Medicare Payment? List the Type field and copy the explanation of this field.

    Payment Code: MEDCAR; Type field: I; Explanation of Type field: P-Patient, I-Insurance, PW-Patient Write Off, IW-Insurance Write off.

    The explanation is listed at the bottom of your screen when the cursor is positioned at the Type field.

6. Write the diagnostic code for Vaginitis.

    616.10

7. How many diagnostic codes do you have in the Master File?

     19

8. How many providers do you have in the practice?

     1

9. What is the TOS code for Consultation?

     3

10. What Master File is Aetna Insurance Co. found in?

     Insurance Company Master File

Chapter 2: Database Entry and Report Writing

NOTE: Students should not use their textbooks for this exercise; they may only use their computers! The audits should be timed. To make it more difficult, you may allow 10 minutes for the audit. The first audit may take longer.

Suggested Time Limit: 15 to 20 minutes

1. What is the amount charged for CPT code 99222?

    $120.00

2. Who is the contact person for the insurance company, Physicians Health Plan?

    Sophie Block

3. What is the Type of Service Code for Diagnostic Laboratory?

    5

4. What is the tax ID# for referring provider Vickie Gylys-Morin, M.D.?

    52-1099432

5. What is the description for CPT Code 45330?

    Sigmoidoscopy, Flexible, Diagnostic

6. What is the address for Toledo Hospital, which is one place your practice uses to treat patients?

    1232 N. Cove Blvd., Toledo, OH 43604

7. What is the diagnosis code for Annual Pelvic Exam, Pap?

    V72.3

8. What are the codes for the six forms of payment accepted by your practice?

    BLCRO, CASH, CHECK, CREDIT, INSURA, and MEDCAR

9. What is the Accounting Code for Adjustment, Error Correction?

    ADJUST

10. How many ICD-9 Diagnostic Codes are entered in your files?

    19

Chapter 3 Patients and Guarantors

Suggested Time Limit: 15 minutes

1. List the passwords acceptable to PM.

    BU, PM, STU

    *This information can be obtained by accessing the Master File menu;
    Passwords; Password Security Master File*

2. What does code 3 in the Billing Cycle Master file indicate?

    Bill Third Week of Every Month.

3. List the four codes you have previously entered in the Financial Class Master File.

    CASH, GOVIN, GROUP, INDIV

4. What is Carlos Giovanni's date of birth?

    7/3/31

5. How do you access Patient Options from the Patient Search Screen?

    *From the Master Files menu, select Patients. At the Patient Search screen, press
    F2/Patient Options. This command is listed at the bottom of the Patient Search
    screen.*

6. What is Tom Kinner's home phone?

    (419)842-7696

7. What is the address for Columbia Gas Company, one of your patient's employers?

    110 Water St., Toledo, OH 43600

8. What is the ICD-9 code for Upper Respiratory Infection?

    465.9

9. Who referred Mary Douglas to your practice?

    Code 2, Vickie Gylys-Morin, M.D.

10. What is the description of CPT code 81000?

    Urinalysis

11. Where is Jack Nicklaus employed?

    Code 4, Department of Public Utilities

12. What is Cathy Ramos' social security number?

    889-23-8965

13. What is the Financial class code for "Other Individual Plans?"

    INDIV

14. What is Debbie Conrad's address?

    4663 Northingam Blvd., Toledo, OH 43623

15. What option is accessed to review the account setup for Billing Data and Insurance Template?

    Patient Options

Chapter 4: Insurance and Day Sheet

1. What is the accounts receivable for Day Sheet 1?

   $5445.00

2. What two menu must you select from the Main Menu to display *Reporting Criteria* dates of the Day Sheets/Deposit Slips?

   There are two options to display Reporting Criteria dates of the Day Sheets/Deposit Slips: select Daily Entry menu; Day Sheet or Daily Entry menu; Daily Deposit Slip

3. From the Day Sheet menu, what is the main heading that displays the day sheets/deposit slips on file and Reporting Criteria?

   DAILY BALANCING SHEET

4. a. List the date(s) of the open day sheet(s). b. List the date(s) of the closed day sheet(s).

   a)   Date of open day sheet: xx/03/xx

   b)   Dates of closed day sheets: xx/01/xx and xx/02/xx

5. To print a deposit slip for Day Sheet 2, what dates must you key at the *Reporting Criteria* block?

   xx/02/xx

6. How many Blue Cross Payments were posted on day sheet xx/02/xx? Where would you find this data?

   Six Blue Cross payments were posted. The Daily Entry and Deposit Slip options provide the data when the date xx/02/xx is entered. The sixth payment is listed on Day Sheet, page 2.

7. What is the account balance for Tom Kinner?

   $130.00

   The amount can be obtained in two ways:
   Patients; Patients Search Screen; V/View or
   Update Transactions; F4/Account Summary

8. What Financial Class is Jack Nicklaus?

    INDIV

9. What is the Referring Physician code for Mary Douglas?

    #2

10. What amount did Blue Cross reimburse for Carlos Giovanni on xx/02/xx?

    $420.00

11. What is the description for ICD-9 code 285.9?

    Anemia

12. What is the tax ID# for Kathreen Simon, M.D., one of your referring providers?

    47-295876

13. Which option on the main menu allows you to print a listing of all patients?

    Reports

14. What does the Financial Class code **GOVIN** represent?

    Government-Sponsored Insurance Program

15. Where would you go to display complete transaction information on CONDEB's account when she inquires about her account on the telephone?

    Daily Entry menu; Update Transactions; F4/Account Summary.

    You would not choose Master Files menu; Patients; Patient Search screen because this screen does not display the insurance write offs.

Chapter 5: New Patients and Day Sheet

1. What is the account balance for Carlos Giovanni?

    $700.00

    This information is available in two places: Daily Entry menu; Update Transactions; F4/Account Summary or Master Files menu; Patient Search screen, V/view.

2. What is the <u>total amount</u> of write off charges for John Thomas?

    $20

    This information is available from the Daily Entry menu; Update Transactions.

3. What procedure code was charged to Tom Kinner on Day 3?

    99213

    Select Daily Entry menu; Day sheet 3; abstract the procedure code charged to Tom Kinner.

4. What is the total write-off charges for Day 2?

    $140

    Select the Daily Entry Menu and key XX/02/XX twice. Press M for More to display all pages of the day sheet. The write-off charges as the total amount listed in the Adjustment column

5. What three patients were credited with insurance payments on Day 3 and what is the total of the three payments?

    John Thomas, Carlos Giovanni, and Tom Kinner. The total payment was $291.00.

    Select Daily Entry menu; Deposit Slip or Day Sheet; Enter the date for Day 3; abstract the information from Day Sheet 3. The total payment is listed on Day Sheet 3, page 2.

6. What is Rosa Jackson's birthdate?

    08/21/90

7. Who is David Michael's employer?

   #3, Columbia Gas Co.

8. Who referred Helen Gunn to your practice?

   #1, William Knopp, M.D.

9. Who is the secondary carrier for David Michaels?

   #4, Physicians Health Plan

10. What is Rosa Jackson's relationship to her guarantor?

    CH (child)

11. Print a detailed group report for patients with the last name from L to Z.

    DETAILED GROUP REPORT FOR PATIENTS WITH THE LAST NAME FROM L TO Z:

YOUR MEDICAL CLINIC   **Page: 1**

Patient Grouping Report
Ordered By: Patient Account #
Account # Range: L through Z

Account #	Name:	Provider	Guar #1	Guar#2	Phone
MICDAV	**Michaels, David**	1		0	(419)474-8862
MICLIS	**Michaels, Lisa**	1		0	(419)474-8862
NICJAC	**Nicklaus, Jack**	1		0	(419)536-8888
RAMCAT	**Ramos, Cathy**	1		0	(419)633-5840
THOJOH	**Thomas, John**	1		0	(419)866-9220

Total Number of Patients Listed: 5

The detailed group report is generated as follows: Reports menu; Patient Listings; Grouping; Range: L through Z; Summary Listing; Printer; Report Listing

12. What is the BLCRO amount posted to CONDEB's account?

    $210

    Select Daily Entry menu; Update Transactions; F4/Account or bring up the Balance Sheet and abstract the BLCRO payment.

Chapter 6: Appointment Scheduler

1. List the total charges for Day Sheet 4.

    $427.00

2. List the Other Insurance Payments and Medicare Payment codes.

    Payment Code Master File:
    Other Insurance Payments, INSURA; Medicare Payment, MEDCAR

3. List the diagnostic code for a headache and a cough.

    Diagnosis Code Master File:
    Headache 784.0; Cough 786.2

4. a. Index Scheduling Files.
    b. From the Main Calendar screen, list the options you selected to Index Scheduling Files.

    Main Calendar screen:
    Utilities; Index Scheduling Files; Index

5. a. Build three Appointment Screens.
    b. From the Main Calendar screen, list the options you selected to Build three Appointment Screens.

    Main Calendar screen:
    Utilities; Build Appointment Screens; Key a 3 and press Enter

6. Schedule appointments for two new patients, Gail Roberts 10:00 to 10:30 AM, and John Crotz 10:30 to 11:00 AM for a Hx & Phys. When you are finished, generate a print screen of your Daily Appointment Scheduling screen.

DAILY APPOINTMENT SCHEDULING SCREEN:

```
*********************************************************************
xx/xx/xx P 1
*********************************************************************
10:00 A.M.  ROBGAI
10:15 A.M.  ROBGAI
10:30 A.M.  CROJOH
10:45 A.M.  CROJOH
11:00 A.M.
11:15 A.M.
11:30 A.M. LUNCH
12:00 P.M. LUNCH
12:15 P.M. LUNCH
12:30 P.M. LUNCH
12:45 P.M. LUNCH
 1:00 P.M.
 1:15 P.M.
 1:30 P.M.
 1:45 P.M.
 2:00 P.M.
 2:15 P.M.
 2:30 P.M.
*********************************************************************
XXXXX   ( ) Menu   ( ) View   ( ) Name   ( ) Search   ( ) Help   ( )Return
*********************************************************************
```

7. From the Reports menu, select the Daily/Weekly/Monthly Schedule. Then print a Daily Schedule/Summary Report for Gail Roberts and John Crotz.

DAILY SCHEDULE/SUMMARY REPORT:

Page: 1

Daily/Weekly/Monthly Summary Schedule
xx/xx/xx Provider: 1   Excluding Meetings
Excluding: Sunday Saturday

Date	Time:	Length (Min)	Prov:	Fac:	Type:	Comment:
ROBGAI##	*Name not Found*					
xx/xx/xx	*10:00 AM*	*30*	*1*		*NEWPAT*	*History & Physical*
CROJOH##	*Name not Found*					
xx/xx/xx	*10:30 AM*	*30*	*1*		*NEWPAT*	*History & Physical*

8. From the Main Calendar screen, list the options you would select to print a single route slip.

> *Main Calendar screen:*
> *Reports; Route Slips; Single Route Slip*

9. List the two codes and charges for Helen Gunn on Day Sheet 4.

> *99213 $45.00; 93000 $85.00*

10. List Jack Nicklaus' account balance.

> *$445*
>
> *The amount can be obtained in two ways:*
> *Patients; Patients Search Screen; V/View or*
> *Update Transactions; F4/Account Summary*

Chapter 9: Billing and Practice Management

1. List the total adjustments of your last day sheet.

    17.00 CR

2. List the total amount deposited in the bank from your last day sheet/deposit slip.

    $382.00

3. List the description for Type of Service Codes 1, 2, and 3.

    1 Medical Care; 2 Surgery, 3 Consultation

4. What is the current amount due on John Thomas' account?

    $380

    The amount can be obtained in two ways:
    Patients; Patients Search Screen; V/View or
    Update Transactions; F4/Account Summary

5. List the menus and/or options you would follow to print statements.

    - *Daily Entry Menu*
    - *Statements*
    - *White Paper--PgDn*
    - *Patient Statements (Statement Dunning Messages)—PgDn*
    - *Select either Save or Return without Saving*
    - *Printer*

6. Change Cathy Ramos' print status from PRNTD to NOTPRNTD. List the options you would follow to do so.

    - *Insurance Menu*
    - *Highlight RAMCAT at the Scan All Insurance Forms screen*
    - *Press E/Edit*
    - *From the Insurance Form# screen, scroll to Print, and press Enter*
    - *From the Insurance Form Print pop-up menu, press Entr to select ( ) Change Print Status*
    - *At the highlighted (·) NOT PRNTD option, press Enter to engage the Not Prntd status*

7. Once you change the system date to approximately 2 months past the current date that is listed, even if it is past the current year, list the options and/or menus you would follow to print an Aged Accounts Receivable Report.

    - *Report Menu*
    - *End of Month option*
    - *Aged Accounts Receivable (Pop-up screen)*
    - *( ) Yes, Age Accounts*

8. Display the End of Month; Charged/Paid Report; Summary Listing on your monitor. What are the total charges listed in the report?

    $6,177

9. What is the total Insurance Payments Applied, including the insurance payments percentage shown on the previous Charged/Paid Report—Summary Listing .

    Insurance Payments Applied: $1,290, 25.57%

10. List the menus and/or options you must follow to access the Productivity/Analysis Report.

    Reports Menu
    End of Month
    Production Analysis

CHAPTER TESTS

For each chapter, a set of multiple choice and true/false questions, including the correct answers are included in this section. The same test questions are contained in the F. A. Davis CyberTest™ test-generating program, which is available to adopters of the textbook. The test bank is based on the end-of-chapter review questions in the textbook, and computer audits, which in turn are based on the student objectives. CyberTest™ also permits you to add your own questions or modify those in the test bank.

Chapter 1: Developing Computer Competency

Multiple Choice: Select the best answer.

1. A collection of related files that serve as a base for retrieving information
   a. volatile
   b. database
   c. execute
   d. auxiliary
   e. boot up

Answer: b

2. The process of turning on a computer system
   a. volatile
   b. execute
   c. database
   d. boot up
   e. auxiliary

Answer: d

3. To carry out a program's instructions
   a. execute
   b. boot up
   c. volatile
   d. auxiliary
   e. database

Answer: a

4. Additional or supplementary
   a. database
   b. auxiliary
   c. execute
   d. boot up
   e. b and d

Answer: b

5. Memory device that loses information when the power is turned off
   a. computer chip
   b. CPU
   c. speakers
   d. volatile
   e. a and d

Answer: d

6. Cue on the monitor
   a. escape key
   b. menu
   c. prompt
   d. a and b
   e. none of the above

Answer: c

7. A hard copy refers to
   a. output from a laser printer only
   b. a document used for interoffice purposes only
   c. output from a dot matrix printer only
   d. output from any computer's printer
   e. a copy that cannot be scratched or defaced

Answer: d

8. A small- or medium-sized computer
   a. computer without sound
   b. mainframe
   c. minicomputer
   d. supermicro
   e. computer without CDROM

Answer: c

9. The most common way to input data is through
   a. pointing device
   b. a scanning device
   c. voice-input devices
   d. keyboard
   e. a mouse

Answer: d

10. The device that translates computer signals to telephone signals is a:
    a. modem
    b. CDROM
    c. fax
    d. a and c
    e. a and b

Answer: a

11. Storage device that has greater storage capacity than a floppy disk
    a. CD-ROM
    b. auxiliary floppies
    c. CPU
    d. a and b
    e. b and c

Answer: a

12. A FAX machine
    a. includes hardware that tells the computer how to process data
    b. transmits graphics or documents via telephone lines
    c. is used primarily as an output device
    d. a and c
    e. b and c

Answer: b

13. Formatting a disk
    a. erases all files on a disk
    b. partitions a disk into a series of concentric tracks
    c. partitions a disk into sectors
    d. b and c
    e. all of the above

Answer: e

14. The part of a computer system that controls and monitors the system is:
    a. the central processing unit (CPU)
    b. the disk storage unit
    c. RAM
    d. the controller
    e. auxiliary devices

Answer: a

15. The process of initializing a new disk is called
    a. backing up
    b. formatting
    c. booting
    d. diskcopy
    e. a and d

Answer: b

16. The order of computers from smallest to largest is
    a. mainframe, mini, and micro
    b. micro, mini, and mainframe
    c. mini, micro, and mainframe
    d. mainframe, micro, and mini
    e. b and c

Answer: b

17. The storage device on a micro is generally
    a. floppy drive
    b. hard drive
    c. CPU
    d. a and b
    e. all of the above

Answer: d

18. Which of the following would not be considered a computer hardware device?
    a. a monitor
    b. a keyboard
    c. a disk operating system (DOS)
    d. a disk drive
    e. all of the above

Answer: c

19 The most common and inexpensive printer for a personal computer is a
    a. daisy-wheel printer
    b. laser printer
    c. dot-matrix printer
    d. ink-jet printer
    e. typewriter that functions as a printer

Answer: c

20. Which of the following is NOT a hardware component of a typical computer system?
    a. a display screen
    b. a printer
    c. the CPU
    d. a disk drive
    e. a, c, and d only

Answer: b

21. Which of the following is true concerning computers?
    a. to use computers effectively requires no training
    b. computers require no maintenance
    c. an understanding of basic principles plus hands-on experience is necessary to use computer programs effectively
    d. a and b
    e. b and c

Answer: c

22. Which of the following is not a feature found on keyboards?
    a. numeric keypad
    b. function keys
    c. return key
    d. NumLock key
    e. none of the above

Answer: e

23. Repetitive strain injury (RSI) accounts for
    a. about 10% of job-related illnesses
    b. about 15% of job-related illnesses
    c. about 80% of job-related illnesses
    d. over half of all job-related illnesses
    e. none of the above

Answer: d

True/False

24. Mainframes are the largest, fastest, most powerful, and most expensive computers.

Answer: T

25. The return key is also called the enter key.

Answer: T

26. Every microcomputer has three types of memory that are known as RAM, ROM, and DOS.

Answer: F

27. Some microcomputers are not designed to work with monitors.

Answer: F

28. Random-access memory (RAM) is volatile, and data stored in it disappear when the computer's power is turned off.

Answer: T

29. The best way to keep your floppy disk clean is to wipe the exposed surface with a clean tissue.

Answer: F

30. It is not necessary to format a new disk if you plan to use it as a backup disk.

Answer: F

31. The read/write head in a disk drive writes and reads data by sensing a trail of magnetic variations on the diskette.

Answer: T

32. To avoid RSI, relax your shoulders and keep them level.

Answer: T

33. It is important to wait until the CPU completes the processing before you strike any keys.

Answer: T

34 To understand how a computer program is designed, you do not have to practice the various features.

Answer: F

35. A positive attitude helps you become successful in achieving the objectives of each chapter.

Answer: T

Chapter 2: Database Entry and Report Printing

Multiple Choice: Select the best answer.

1. Stores medical diagnoses commonly used in a medical practice
   a. Facility Master File
   b. Provider Master File
   c. Diagnosis Code Master File
   d. Payment Code Master File
   e. Charge Code Master File

Answer: c

2. Contains information on all of the outside facilities you send your patients to for services
   a. Provider Master File
   b. Facility Master File
   c. Diagnosis Code Master File
   d. Payment Code Master File
   e. Charge Code Master File

Answer: b

3. Stores payment codes that apply a credit to an account
   a. Payment Code Master File
   b. Facility Master File
   c. Provider Master File
   d. Diagnosis Code Master File
   e. Charge Code Master File

Answer: a

4. Contains information needed to produce insurance forms for each physician in your practice
   a. Facility Master File
   b. Provider Master File
   c. Diagnosis Code Master File
   d. Payment Code Master File
   e. Charge Code Master File

Answer: b

5. Stores accounting codes and CPT codes
    a. Provider Master File
    b. Facility Master File
    c. Diagnosis Code Master File
    d. Payment Code Master File
    e. Charge Code Master File

Answer: e

6. Five-digit codes that correspond to accepted classifications of diseases and medical conditions.
    a. CPT
    b. ICD-9
    c. modifiers
    d. both a and b
    e. b and c

Answer: b

7. List of commands that appear from a menu bar at the bottom of a screen.
    a. Save
    b. Edit
    c. Cancel or Delete
    d. Add
    e. all of the above

Answer: e

8. Two-digit codes that describe a specific variation from a normal medical service or procedure are:
    a. CPT codes with a suffix
    b. codes with a suffix
    c. both a and b
    d. modifiers
    e. none of the above

Answer: d

9. To change information in an ICD-9 code file, you would
    a. delete the file
    b. add a file
    c. edit the file
    d. a and b
    e. all of the above

Answer: c

10. To exit PM and sign off the system, you must choose the following selection at the main menu screen.
    a. Daily Entry
    b. Quit
    c. Insurance
    d. Reports
    e. Utilities

Answer: b

11. Medical care, surgery, consultation, assistance to surgery, and diagnostic interpretation are code descriptions found in the Master File relating to:
    a. payment of service
    b. place of service
    c. type of service
    d. a and c only
    e. of the above

Answer: c

12. To retrieve a stored code file, highlight the code and press the following key or command:
    a. C
    b. E
    c. M
    d. PR
    e. b and c

Answer: b

13. CASH, CREDIT, and BLCRO are codes found in the
    a. Diagnostic Code File
    b. Referring Provider File
    c. Charge Code File
    d. Insurance Company File
    e. Payment Code Master File

Answer: e

True/False

14. The escape key takes you to the end of a file.

Answer: F

15. Data can become corrupted or lost if PM program is not signed off properly.

Answer: T

16. The menu bar at the bottom of the screen lists available commands that allow you to complete various program functions.

Answer: T

17. The Master Files menu is where all reports are generated.

Answer: F

18. The Reports Menu prints reports but is not a useful tool in the management of a medical practice.

Answer: F

19. The **hot key** can be pressed for immediate access to a menu or file.

Answer: T

20. The Charge Code Master File stores accounting codes.

Answer: T

Chapter 3: Patients and Guarantors

Multiple Choice: Select the best answer.

1. The Company Master File stores
   a. the company address that the medical practice bills under
   b. all the insurance companies used by patients
   c. the name of the medical practice
   d. a and c
   e. b and c

Answer: d

2. The *Clear Disk Space* feature performs the function of:
   a. adding files
   b. permanently erasing information from the hard drive
   c. indexes files
   d. a and b
   e. b and c

Answer: e

3. To review or edit the Account Setup File or the Insurance Template File after it has been saved, press the following key at the Patient Search File:
   a. F1
   b. F2
   c. F3
   d. enter
   e. return

Answer: b

4. If you do not know the required code to be entered in a field and need to access the Master File directly, enter the following symbol at the appropriate field:
   a. a slash
   b. an explanation mark
   c. a question mark
   d. an asterisk
   e. an equal sign

Answer: c

5. The guarantor figures that you display on your monitor must match
   a. the guarantor figures shown in the database
   b. the guarantor figures shown in the billing data
   c. the guarantor figures shown on the insurance template
   d. b and c only
   e. none of the above

Answer: e

6. The majority of patients in your office are set up in the billing data section of the Patient Setup file with:
   a. An Open Item account code designated as O
   b. A Balance Forward account code designated as B
   c. A Credit account code designated as C
   d. a and c
   e. b and c

Answer: a

7. The one who is ultimately responsible for all charges on an account.
   a. patient
   b. fiscal agent
   c. insurance carrier
   d. guarantor
   e. spouse

Answer: d

8. Patient's vital statistics, i.e., address, phone number, and birthdate consist of
   a. insurance template
   b. financial class requirements
   c. demographic
   d. both a and b
   e. both b and c

Answer: c

9. Open-item accounting posts payments
   a. to the first charge that was incurred on the account regardless if that check applied to the charge
   b. to the last charge that was incurred on the account regardless if that check applied to the charge
   c. to the total balance on the account as a continuous posting procedure
   d. to specific charges
   e. to governmental guidelines

Answer: d

10. Balance forward accounting posts payments to:
    a. the first charge that was incurred on the account regardless if that check applied to the charge
    b. the last charge that was incurred on the account regardless if that check applied to the charge
    c. the total balance on the account as a continuous posting procedure
    d. posts payments to specific charges
    e. posts payments according to governmental guidelines

Answer: c

True/False

11. Interrupting the printing of reports may create a critical error. The monitor may display an error message on the monitor.

Answer: T

12. Once a patient's account number has been assigned and saved, it cannot be changed.

Answer: T

13. The guarantor and the patient may be the same person.

Answer: T

14. In PM, your practice has three providers, therefore, always use code 3 for the primary provider.

Answer: F

15. The insurance template stores answers to the questions at the top of an insurance form and allows each patient to have their own template.

Answer: T

Chapter 4: Insurance and Day Sheet Management

Multiple Choice: Select the best answer.

1. The accounting procedure used by PM in which payments are posted with no regard to the charges that they are for is called
   a. balance forward
   b. closed item
   c. open item
   d. a and c
   e. none of the above

Answer: a

2. An advantage to open-item accounting is
   a. flexibility of posting payments to specific charges
   b. a continuous posting procedure
   c. line by line detail of all transactions
   d. a and c
   e. all of the above

Answer: d

3. Payments from patients are entered from the following option of the Daily Entry menu:
   a. credits
   b. payments
   c. daily deposit slip
   d. statements
   e. posttransactions

Answer: e

4. A patient's routing slip can include
   a. procedures performed
   b. services performed
   c. laboratory tests performed
   d. a diagnostic code
   e. all of the above

Answer: e

5. It is necessary to create a backup of your files because
    a. it provides a duplicate copy in case the master disk is corrupted
    b. it provides you with a hard copy to verify entries
    c. it provides a duplicate copy in case of fire
    d. a and c
    e. a and b

Answer: d

6. A responsible party is
    a. always the patient
    b. the party ultimately responsible for any charges
    c. not responsible for the charges if the patient is the legal age of 16 years
    d. a and c
    e. none of the above

Answer: b

7. A third-party payer is the
    a. insurance carrier
    b. dependent who is responsible for the bill
    c. parent or guardian who is responsible for the bill
    d. patient, if there is no insurance policy
    e. none of the above

Answer: a

8. What is the purpose of the Clear Disk Space option on the Utilities menu?
    a. re-index files on the hard drive
    b. temporarily remove files on the hard drive
    c. permanently removes data from the hard drive
    d. a and c
    e. a and b

Answer: d

9. Name the statement that is sent from an insurance carrier to a patient that explains what benefits were paid or excluded from an insurance claim.
    a. billing statement
    b. insurance statement
    c. explanation of benefits (EOB)
    d. a and c
    e. none of the above

Answer: c

10. The deposit slip lists all the payments that will be
    a. credited to patients accounts
    b. entered in the transaction entry screen
    c. deposited in the bank
    d. a and b only
    e. b and c only

Answer: c

11. Open-item billing is required for Medicare patients because
    a. the medical practice is not allowed to send Medicare patients a statement until Medicare pays their allowed charges
    b. the provider is not allowed to bill Medicare patients for their services
    c. it prevents the bill being sent to a patient until Medicare reimburses the office
    d. a and c
    e. all of the above

Answer: d

12. When a provider is willing to adjust a disallowed portion of an insurance claim, the office will
    a. debit the amount to bad debts
    b. write-off the amount
    c. debit the amount to the patients' account
    d. send a bill to the guarantor
    e. none of the above

Answer: b

13. A physician who accepts assignment
    a. assigns the bill to a collection agency
    b. accepts whatever the fiscal intermediary sends in as full payment of the patients' bill minus the deductible and copayment
    c. accepts whatever the fiscal intermediary sends in as full payment
    d. a and c
    e. none of the above

Answer: b

14. Charges and payments are posted to accounts in the
    a. account setup
    b. insurance accounts
    c. statements file
    d. transaction entry
    e. a and c only

Answer: d

15. The key at the Transaction Entry screen that allows you to display the totals for your current posting session.
    a. F4
    b. Escape
    c. Update
    d. Both a and b
    e. a, b, and c

Answer: a

True/False

16. The F2 key accesses the insurance template file.

Answer: T

17. To go to the end of a file, press PgDn.

Answer: T

18. A disadvantage of open-time accounting is that it does not provide flexibility of posting payments to specific charges.

Answer: F

19. When the physician accepts assignment, the insurance carrier sends the check to the patient.

Answer: F

20. To edit a Dx Code on the Transaction Entry screen, press F3 when the cursor is positioned at the DX Code: field.

Answer: T

Chapter 5: New Patients and Day Sheet Management

Multiple Choice: Select the best answer.

1. Information on the patient registration form includes:
    a. place of employment
    b. medical services
    c. mailing address
    d. a and c
    e. all of the above

Answer: d

2. What provision ensures that a patient is not reimbursed more than 100% of their total medical expenses?
    a. invoice
    b. coordination of benefits (COB)
    c. superbill
    d. walk-out statement
    e. none of the above

Answer: b

3. An insurance carrier allows $30 of a $50 fee charged to a patient. If the doctor accepts assignment, the $20 difference above the allowable charge is the
    a. write off
    b. tax deductible
    c. the difference between the charged and allowed amount
    d. the amount the patient must pay
    e. both a and c

Answer: e

4. Which of the following statements is true concerning coordination of benefits?
    a. an individual policy is primary over a group policy
    b. the husband's policy is primary to the wife's
    c. Medicare is always the secondary payer
    d. the primary carrier takes into account benefits that are payable by the secondary carrier
    e. supplemental insurance is always primary

Answer: d

5. The accounting system used for Medicare patients is called:
   a. balance-forward billing
   b. closed-item billing
   c. open-item billing
   d. credit-item billing
   e. a and c

Answer: c

6. If you are not in balance on your current active day sheet and need to edit it, select the following option:
   a. daily deposit slips
   b. statements
   c. route slips
   d. post transactions
   e. update transactions

Answer: e

7 The superbill is used to
   a. attach to the insurance claim form for reimbursement purposes
   b. serve as a receipt of medical services performed
   c. serve as a record of services with CPT and ICD-9 coding
   d. a and c
   e. all of the above

Answer: e

8. To edit a transaction on a closed day sheet, you must
   a. make an adjustment on a subsequent day sheet
   b. change the date back to previous day and make adjustment
   c. make adjustments at the end of the month
   d. record errors in the responsible party's account
   e. correct errors on the detailed active day sheet report

Answer: a

9. When can a walk-out receipts be printed?
   a. at the end of the month
   b. after you are finished posting the payment transactions for the patient
   c. after the day sheet is closed
   d. before the patient sees the physician
   e. none of the above

Answer: b

True/False

10. Generally, when a patient has secondary insurance, the primary carrier is billed first.

Answer: T

11. After entering data on a screen, always press the return key to display appropriate commands to continue.

Answer: F

12. Medicare patients cannot be billed until payment from Medicare is received.

Answer: T

13. Cash flow refers to checks and cash received by the medical practice.

Answer: T

14. Balance forward transactions are monies owed to the patients.

Answer: F

15. When a patient has two insurance policies, you always bill the secondary carrier first.

Answer: F

Chapter 6: Appointment Scheduler

Multiple Choice: Select the best answer.

1. Two important daily housekeeping tasks in the Appointment Scheduler are building appointment screens and indexing files. These programs are accessed from the Appointment Scheduler's
   a. Clear Disk Space option
   b. Appointment Type Master File
   c. Utilities Menu
   d. Daily/Weekly/Monthly Schedule
   e. Both a and c

Answer: c

2. The appointment scheduler can be accessed from the Daily Entry menu by
   a. selecting the Scheduler option
   b. selecting Master Files
   c. selecting Post Transactions option
   d. a and c
   e. all of the above

Answer: d

3. If an error message appears on the screen while you are working in any part of the Appointment Scheduler, you need to:
   a. access the Utilities option
   b. sign off PM
   c. index the Scheduling Files
   d. a and c
   e. all of the above

Answer: d

4. The PM route slip can be used to:
   a. act as an encounter form
   b. replace the super bill
   c. inform the front desk of all services
   d. record the patient's diagnosis and CPT procedures that were performed during the office visit
   e. all of the above

Answer: e

5. The New Patient List is used as
    a. a reminder to complete the patient file
    b. a reminder to complete the guarantor file
    c. a reminder to send statements
    d. a reminder to call the patient
    e. a and b only

Answer: e

6. The "?" is used to determine the
    a. patient account #
    b. appointment type
    c. CPT code
    d. a and b only
    e. all of the above

Answer: e

7. A blinking highlighted date displayed on the Main Calendar indicates
    a. an error
    b. the prior working day date
    c. the current date
    d. subsequent working day date
    e. none of the above

Answer: c

8. The Daily Appointment Summary Schedule designates new patients with
    a. an asterisk
    b. double pound sign
    c. an exclamation mark
    d. a percent sign
    e. a dollar sign

Answer: b

9. The standard claim form accepted by most insurance carriers and governmental fiscal agents
    is the
    a. route slip
    b. encounter form
    c. patient statement
    d. HCFA 1000
    e. HCFA 1500

Answer: e

10. The following two locations in the Daily Entry Menu provide access to the Appointment Scheduler:
    a. from the Post Transaction screen
    b. by pressing F4 at the Guarantor screen
    c. from the Scheduler option
    d. a and c
    e. a and b

Answer: d

11. When a physician operates on a fixed appointment schedule and a person arrives without an appointment, requesting to see the doctor, you should probably:
    a. send the patient away
    b. send the patient to another physician
    c. tell the patient you will call them as soon as you have a cancellation
    d. ask the patient to come back the first thing the following morning
    e. try to squeeze the patient in for a brief visit and let the doctor decide what the next step should be

Answer: e

12. To cancel a stored appointment, you must select the following option:
    a. cancel and edit
    b. detail and delete
    c. edit and cancel
    d. both a and b
    e. none of the above

Answer: b

13. The appointment scheduler should be:
    a. checked over at least once a week
    b. checked upon the arrival of each patient
    c. checked at least every 30 minutes
    d. treated as a confidential record
    e. both b and d

Answer: e

14. Every effort should be made to arrange an appointment time that is satisfactory for the patient because:
    a. the doctor's time is not of primary importance
    b. the patient should be made to feel the doctor wants to see him or her
    c. emergencies are handled at the end of the day
    d. "no-shows" are costly
    e. a, b, and d

Answer: b

15. One method that can be used to allow time to catch-up, should the appointments begin falling behind schedule, is:
    a. to limit the number of patients seen per day
    b. to see patients on a double-booked basis
    c. to take shorter lunch-breaks
    d. to leave a 15- or 20-minute interval free late in the afternoon
    e. cancel those afternoon appointments that you know the doctor will not have time for

Answer: d

16. If a patient calls to cancel an appointment, you should:
    a. reprimand him or her sternly
    b. have the patient speak with the doctor
    c. express regret
    d. immediately offer a new appointment time
    e. all of the above

Answer: d

17. If the doctor calls you and explains that he or she will be delayed in arriving at the office, the best approach to this problem is to:
    a. cancel all the appointments and re-schedule them for another day
    b. tell the patients that there will be a long wait
    c. explain the delay and give the patients a choice of either waiting or re-scheduling their appointments for another day
    d. tell the patients nothing, but make sure there are plenty of magazines for everyone to read
    e. either a or b

Answer: c

True/False Questions

18. You can only book appointments in the current and subsequent months using PM.

Answer: T

19. If you schedule an appointment in a prior month, a critical error will result.

Answer: T

20. PM does not check to see if there are any conflicts or double bookings with the appointment you schedule.

Answer: F

21. The Daily Appointment Schedule is usually produced 2 days before the scheduled appointments so the physician can review them.

Answer: F

22. The same procedure is used to edit a 15-minute and a 30-minute appointment.

Answer: F

23. A patient who has a 30-minute appointment takes up two blocks of time on the appointment scheduler

Answer: T

24. On the Daily Appointment Summary Schedule, new patients are designated by two ** after their patient account numbers.

Answer: F

25. The Reports option of the Main Calendar only allows you to print a report, but you cannot view it on the screen.

Answer: F

Chapter 7: Billing and Collections

Multiple Choice: Select the best answer.

1. The office policy to extend credit to individual patients is usually determined by
   a. the office manager
   b. a credit agency
   c. the office manager
   d. a bank
   e. the physician

Answer: e

2. Who is usually responsible for informing patients of an office policy that states, "payment is expected at the time of service?"
   a. the doctor
   b. the accountant
   c. the office manager
   d. the insurance company
   e. a and c

Answer: c

3. If a bill is turned over to a collection agency
   a. the office staff and the collection agency both work together to collect payment
   b. the collection agency usually requests that the patient make payment to the doctor
   c. the collection agency will have access to the patient's medical record to assist in the collection process
   d. the patient will be requested to make payment to the collection agency.
   e. c and d

Answer: d

4. Even if a Medicare claim is pending, a patient with an outstanding balance should
   a. not be billed until the insurance carrier pays the bill
   b. continue to be billed each month
   c. have the balance written off the account
   d. consult the doctor about the bill
   e. a and c

Answer: a

5. For the physician's office, the use of a collection agency represents
    a. an efficient mechanism for collecting debts
    b. a "last resort" to collect the bill
    c. a helper in office collections
    d. a means for collecting at least 20% of overdue bills
    e. a normal method to collect bills that are 60 days past due

Answer: b

6. The amount of money that the doctor charges patients for services rendered is NOT considered a/an
    a. income
    b. earnings
    c. profit
    d. charge
    e. accounts receivable

Answer: c

7. Patients who pay cash for office calls should:
    a. be given a discount
    b. be encouraged to pay by check
    c. given a walk-out receipt
    d. be informed that they will receive a statement at the end of the month
    e. both a and c

Answer: c

8. Which of the following statements is true?
    a. The ability and willingness of the patient to pay can easily be determined at the first visit.
    b. It is not necessary to age accounts in a small office with few patients.
    c. Every effort should be made to send out monthly statements promptly and on the same date each month.
    d. Accounts receivables never depreciate and so collections should always be pursued.
    e. None of the above.

Answer: c

9. To make it easier for the patient requiring prolonged and expensive care to pay his/her bill, the office might suggest that the patient
    a. pay the bill in cash
    b. take out a bank loan
    c. make a regular monthly or weekly payment of a fixed amount
    d. b and c
    d. none of the above

Answer: c

10. The pegboard system simultaneously generates a
    a. daily earnings summary
    b. deposit slip and ledger card
    c. patient charge and receipt slip
    d. both b and c
    e. all of the above

Answer: e

11. The principal purpose of the day sheet in a computerized office is
    a. the same as that of a pegboard system
    b. less extensive and more complicated than a pegboard system
    c. more extensive and less complicated than a pegboard system
    d. both a and b
    e. both a and c

Answer: a

12. The trend in billing is to send the patient
    a. a copy of his/her ledger card
    b. a copy of the insurance claim
    c. an itemized statement
    d. a walk-out statement
    e. both b and c

Answer: c

13. The collection of accounts can be improved if the office
    a. sends statements on a regular basis
    b. sends statements that are itemized and accurate
    c. has a good follow-up system
    d. all of the above
    e. both a and b

Answer: d

14. If 3 months elapse from the time the first statement is sent and still no payment has been remitted, you should:
    a. send no further bills
    b. place the account with a collection agency
    c. send a threatening letter
    d. tell the patient the doctor will initiate a lawsuit
    e. send a letter with a request for payment

Answer: e

15. Collection trends and necessary follow-up measures in the office can be determined from
    a. the summary of the patients' detail transactions
    b. the local credit bureau
    c. the age analysis account figures
    d. all of the above
    e. both b and c

Answer: c

16. "Aging accounts" refers to:
    a. analyzing the status of accounts payable
    b. analyzing the status of accounts receivable
    c. analyzing the cash flow
    d. all of the above
    e. both b and c

Answer: b

17. If your office receives a call from a patient whose account has been turned over to a collection agency, you should:
    a. ask the patient to bring in a payment immediately to avoid a lawsuit
    b. ask the patient to talk to the physician
    c. tell the patient you will contact the agency to have further collections stopped
    d. explain that the patient must now deal with the agency who is handling the account
    e. both a and d

Answer: d

18. The criteria for selecting a credit agency should be to
    a. select an aggressive company
    b. select an agency that charges less than 15% to collect the bill
    c. select an agency that will go to the patient's home to collect the bill
    d. both a and b
    e. none of the above

Answer: e

19. The Federal Communications Commission statutes govern the use of the telephone for collections and prohibits the following:
    a. repeated calls to the guarantor
    b. calls to neighbors
    c. threatening calls
    d. both b and c
    e. all of the above

Answer: e

20. When a patient and physician enter a bilateral agreement that permits the patient to pay a fee in more than four installments:
    a. the physician is required to orally inform the patient
    b. either the physician or office manager must orally inform the patient
    c. a written disclosure form stating all pertinent information, regardless of the existence of any finance charges, should be given to and signed by the patient
    d. a written disclosure form stating all pertinent information be given to and signed by the patient only if finance charges will be assessed
    e. a copy of the office policy must be given to and signed by the patient

Answer: c

True/False Questions

21. Cash flow refers to checks or cash received by the medical practice.

Answer: T

22. If a bank deposit is over $5000, the doctor usually makes the deposit.

Answer: F

23. Collecting payment at the time of service relieves the office staff of the burden of collection if a patient fails to pay the bill.

Answer: T

24. Computerized billing systems usually do not produce a bank deposit slip.

Answer: F

25. The pegboard system is also known as a triple-entry system.

Answer: F

Chapter 8: Insurance Processing

Multiple Choice: Select the best answer.

1. Before any information on a patient can be given to an insurance company, attorney, or government agent, you must obtain
   a. a payment in full of the patient's account
   b. a check from the insurance company
   c. permission from the patient's attorney
   d. a "release of information" signed by the patient
   e. c and d

Answer: d

2. When filing a claim for an out-of-state patient who is under the Blue Shield reciprocity program, you must:
   a. file the claim with the patient's home plan in his or her state
   b. send the claim to the regional Blue Shield office where the policy originates
   c. bill the local Blue Shield office on the local Blue Shield claim form
   d. bill the local Blue Shield office on the patient's local Blue Shield claim form
   e. either a or b

Answer: e

3. The federal government participates with all states in a health insurance plan for people on welfare known as:
   a. Medicare
   b. Medicaid
   c. CHAMPUS
   d. b and c
   e. all of the above

Answer: b

4. The authorization to release information of a medical claim is signed by the
   a. physician
   b. insurance carrier
   c. patient
   d. office manager
   e. depends on the office policy

Answer: c

5. Which of the following is NOT a type of Workers' Compensation benefit?
   a. permanent disability
   b. rehabilitation benefits
   c. retirement benefits
   d. medical treatment
   e. b and c

Answer: e

6. A standard form for both group and individual insurance claims that is accepted by almost all insurance companies is referred to as form
   a. SSA-1490
   b. DA 1962
   c. Title XVIII
   d. HCFA 1500
   e. MCAID

Answer: d

7. The insurance program authorizing treatment by civilian physicians at the expense of the government for dependents of military personnel is
   a. Medicaid
   b. IPP
   c. Medi-Medi
   d. CHAMPUS
   e. b and d only

Answer: d

8. To guarantee that the patient is eligible for benefits, the office should:
   a. call the insurance carrier when dealing with a new patient
   b. check the patient's insurance identification card to determine the effective date of coverage
   c. interview the patient to determine their eligibility
   d. both a and c
   e. both b and c

Answer: b

9. The amount a patient is required to pay under a health insurance plan before benefits become payable is referred to as:
   a. the deductible
   b. the coinsurance
   c. the non applicable amount
   d. the assignment of benefits
   e. a and c only

Answer: a

10. If a medical insurance policy has a deductible of $50, the
    a. patient has to pay this amount
    b. patient may deduct this amount from the physician's bill
    c. patient does not have to pay the first $50
    d. physician is reimbursed for $50 by the insurance carrier
    e. the patient and insurance carrier split the $50

Answer: a

11. If a physician indicates on a CHAMPUS form that he or she will not accept assignment, this means that the
    a. patient is liable for the entire bill
    b. doctor will accept whatever CHAMPUS sends in full payment of the bill
    c. doctor expects the patient to pay the deductible
    d. all of the above
    e. both b and c

Answer: a

12. If a person is insured along with others who work for the same firm, that type of coverage is known as
    a. a company sponsored insurance
    b. a copayment
    c. a group plan
    d. work-related insurance
    e. coinsurance

Answer: c

13. Which of the following is true of Medicaid?
    a. It is a federal program providing benefits and services throughout the United States
    b. Each state determines its own eligibility guidelines
    c. It is a state medical assistance plan for the indigent
    d. It is a federal program providing uniform benefits throughout the United States
    e. a, b, and c only

Answer: e

14. Identify the government-sponsored insurance plan that allows designated groups of military personnel to receive medical care from a civilian physician when there is no government facility available.
    a. Social Security Plan
    b. Medicare
    c. Medicaid
    d. CHAMPUS
    e. both a and d

Answer: d

15. When a person is injured on the job, they are generally protected against loss of salary and costs related to medical expenses by:
    a. Medicare
    b. Workers' Compensation
    c. Medicaid
    d. CHAMPUS
    e. b, c, and d

Answer: b

16. The law requires physicians to fill out appropriate forms during a designated time period for Workers' Compensation claims, which may include:
    a. a final report
    b. a progress report
    c. an initial report
    d. a and c only
    e. all of the above

Answer: e

17. Most insurance companies process claims
    a. in batches so that several claims might be combined into one check
    b. according to claim numbers
    c. according to regional districts
    d. on a rotation basis to hospitals and physicians office
    e. a, b, and c

Answer: a

18. When an insurance check is issued to the physician, it usually is accompanied by:
    a. a listing of benefits paid to date (LOB)
    b. an explanation of benefits (EOB)
    c. a form that must be sent to the patient (FOB)
    d. both a and b
    e. both b and c

Answer: b

19. The purpose of managed care is to
    a. help the physician cut down on government claim forms
    b. to provide patients with services they need
    c. to provide medical care in a cost effective setting
    d. both a and b
    e. both b and c

Answer: e

20. The following are styles of managed care plans:
    a. HMOs
    b. IPAs
    c. IPPs
    d. all of the above
    e. a and b only

Answer: d

21. The following is true of HMOs:
    a. notification is not required for emergency treatment
    b. notification must usually be given within 24 hours for emergency treatment
    c. to obtain reimbursement, nonemergency care away from home requires authorization
    d. a woman can choose two primary doctors, and Ob/Gyn and a general physician
    e. b, c, and d

Answer: e

22. HMOs are becoming popular for the following reasons:
    a. they provide reimbursement of cosmetic surgery
    b. members pay a fixed fee in advance, regardless of the number of services received
    c. there are no unexpected medical costs
    d. b and c only
    e. all of the above

Answer: d

23. The following is true about the Preferred Provider Organization (PPO):
    a. it is a formal agreement between the patient and doctor to provide medical care
    b. it is a formal agreement amount that certain health care providers use to treat a specific patient population, such as the employees of a union
    c. it provides contracts with specific hospitals or outpatient-care centers for inpatient and outpatient care
    d. the patient may go to a nonparticpating doctor and the medical fee will be fully covered
    e. both b and c

Answer: e

24. When a patient has Medicare and Medicaid, as well as secondary insurance, you would bill:
    a. Medicare and Medicaid first
    b. the private insurance company first
    c. depends on the insurance carrier
    d. both plans simultaneously
    e. both a and c

Answer: b

25. Some of the features of a Major Medical Plan are that
    a. it covers cosmetic surgery
    b. it includes coverage for costs of illness and injury beyond those covered in the basic medical contract
    c. the employer may share the cost of the insurance premium
    d. b and c
    e. it includes hospital precertification

Answer: d

True/False Questions

26. If a patient has a secondary carrier, a copy of the EOB from the primary carrier is not attached to the insurance billing form prepared for the second company.

Answer: F

27. Selecting the wrong CPT code on an insurance claim form will not delay payment if the doctor accepts assignment.

Answer: F

28. The processing time for claims prepared for optical character readers (OCR) is much quicker than those processed manually.

Answer: T

29. Many insurance carriers will reimburse the patient for medical services if they attach a super bill to the claim form.

Answer: T

30. To qualify for Medicare, you must be 60 years or older.

Answer: F

Chapter 9: Billing and Practice Management

Multiple Choice: Select the best answer.

1. Statement are always generated
    a. the 1st week of the month
    b. depends on the medical practice
    c. bimonthly
    d. weekly
    e. after each office visit

Answer: b

2. Statements generated each month are generally sent to:
    a. the insurance company
    b. the guarantor
    c. the patient's employer
    d. a and b
    e. all of the above

Answer: b

3. To enter a payment, you must
    a. be at the Cash Disbursement menu
    b. select Post Transactions
    c. be at the Master Files menu
    d. both a and b
    e. both a and c

Answer: b

4. If the Individual Statement Setup screen displays a **P,** statements will:
    a. display on the screen
    b. print only in batch forms
    c. print either in batches or individual form
    d. both a and c
    e. both a and b

Answer: c

5. Statements to Medicare patients are generated:
    a. each time they make an office visit
    b. at the end of the month
    c. for transactions that have insurance payments posted to them
    d. according to government statutes
    e. c and d only

Answer: e

6. It is a common practice for the office to send the patient:
   a. a copy of the EOB that is attached to the batch payment check
   b. an itemized statement
   c. a copy of the insurance claim form
   d. b and c only
   e. a and b only

Answer: b

7. The following is true about the Generate Forms option of Insurance menu:
   a. it is used to automatically process insurance claim forms
   b. it is completed before claims are printed
   c. it processes transactions in the holding file and assembles them into insurance forms
   d. a and b only
   e. all of the above

Answer: e

8. To enter a charge, you must
   a. be at the Insurance menu
   b. select Post Transactions
   c. be at the Master Files menu
   d. both a and b
   e. both a and c

Answer: b

9. The following is NOT true of the Insurance Transaction Holding File:
   a. it lists the patients' account number
   b. it lists the ICD codes
   c. it lists the CPT codes
   d. it lists the amount of the charge transaction
   e. b and d only

Answer: b

10. To change the status of an insurance form from PRNTD to NOT PRNTD, you must access the following option:
    a. Insurance Transaction Holding File
    b. Scan Forms
    c. Generate Forms
    d. Master Files
    e. either a and b

Answer: b

11. Electronic Claims Transmission (ECT) is currently mandated by federal law:
    a. for all government insurance programs
    b. for Medicare only
    c. for Medicaid only
    d. b and c
    e. none of the above

Answer: e

12. The following reports can be used to produce statistical data for medical research and predicting epidemics:
    a. CPT Reports of procedures performed to determine the patients' disease
    b. Productivity/Analysis Reports
    c. Charge/Paid Reports
    d. a and b
    e. b and c

Answer: b

13. Which of the following statements is true of the Summary/Charge Paid Report
    a. identifies whether the payment was made by a patient or insurance company
    b. identifies whether the credit was a write-off adjustment
    c. can be used in analyzing the monetary trends of the practice
    d. can be used to negotiate managed-care contracts
    e. all of the above

Answer: e

14. Aging accounts refers to:
    a. summarizing how long patients have been treated by your doctor
    b. both c and d
    c. summarizing the bad debts of the practice
    d. analyzing the status of accounts receivable
    e. analyzing the status of accounts payable

Answer: d

15. The Productivity/Analysis Report and Charge/Paid Report can be generated:
    a. on the screen
    b. on a hard copy
    c. from the Transaction Entry screen
    d. a and b
    e. all of the above

Answer: d

True/False Questions

16. To print an individual statement, you must enter the Guarantor number in two places at the Range of Guarantors: field.

Answer: T

17. One of the reasons batch statements will not print is if **P** is listed at the Screen or Printer: field.

Answer: F

18. If an account is over 120 days past due, the current message will print on all statements.

Answer: F

19. Once insurance forms are printed, the Scan All Insurance Forms screen shows the status of every guarantor as NOT PRINTD.

Answer: T

20. Before you close a day sheet, you must verify that it is in balance.

Answer: T

PATRIOT MEDICAL® DOCUMENTATION

Students who learn *Patriot Medical*® will find that the software is similar to other medical office account management systems. Thus, within a very short period of time, they will be able to transfer their competence to any other system. They should have an understanding of computer software documentation manuals that are provided by the software vendor for the purpose of providing the office staff with a reference on how to run various programs. The *Patriot Medical*® *Report Samples* documentation is included to acquaint students with an actual documentation manual. For those instructor's who want additional reports generated, it can be used to develop supplementary advanced activities.

There are many different combinations that can used to generate *Patriot Medical*® reports. Only a few that are most commonly generated in a medical practice have been included. Each report that follows shows the criteria screen that is completed before the report is printed and contains the following:

- the menu used to access a given report
- a brief description of each report and its functionality
- the criteria screen that is completed before a report is printed
- a hard copy of a given report

WRITE TO US

We welcome your reactions to this book, for we would like it to be as useful to you as possible. Write to us in care of:

F.A. Davis Publishing Co.
Allied Health Division
1915 Arch St.
Philadelphia, PA 19103

Barbara A. Gylys, MEd., CMA-A

PATRIOT MEDICAL ®
REPORT SAMPLES

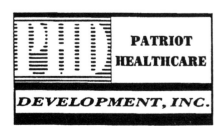

Building Financial Health for your Practice

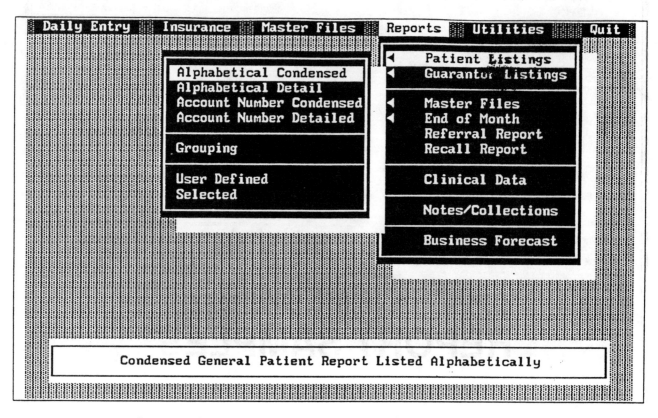

Screen Showing General Patient Listings Available

This is the main menu for the Patient Report section. These menu selections include general patient listings both in condensed and detailed formats, the patient grouping report, the patient user defined report and the selected patient report are also accessed from here.

Reports Shown on the following Pages:

Patient Grouping Report
User Defined Patient Report

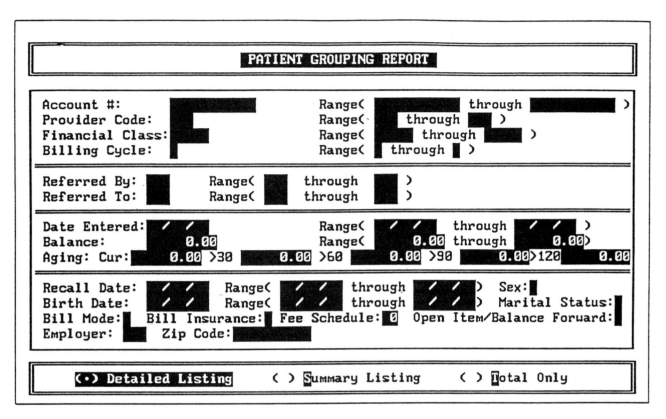

Patient Grouping Criteira Screen

The Patient Grouping allows you to list your patients by any criteria you like. The criteria items encompass all fields related to the patient. This way you can isolate your patient listing to your requirements.

The criteria ranges from Account # to zip code. This report is available in summary, detailed or total only format. Summary lists the patient's Account#, First and Last Name, Primary Provider, Guarantor #1, Guarantor #2 and Phone #. The detailed listing is an extensive listing, displaying all the information about a patient. If you just want the total number of patients that in a given category then you can choose to print reports in the total only format.

Example Shown: Summary Patient Grouping Report for All Patients

Patient Grouping Report

Account #	Name:	Provider	Guar #1	Guar#2	Phone
BURAMA	BURCHNELL,AMANDA	JRN	8	0	(614)852-4951
CREHAU	CREAMER,HAUNS	JRN	7	0	(614)852-0229
DAVJON	DAVIS,JONATHAN	JRN	9	0	(614)852-9649
DAVMAR	DAVIS,MARY	JRN	1	0	(614)852-1933
ELLDOR	ELLIS,DOROTHY	JRN	5	0	(614)874-3492
FREDAW	FREW,DAWN	JRN	2	0	(614)852-4825
GRABET	GRAY,BETTY	JRN	12	0	(614)869-4100
HENWES	HENDERSON,WESLEY	JRN	10	0	(614)869-2797
LAWWIL	LAWSON,WILLIAM	JRN	3	0	(513)834-2065
LEWTER	LEWIS,TERESA	JRN	4	0	(614)852-3408
MONREE	MONROE,REED	JRN	11	0	(513)462-8519
SHIRUS	SHIPE,RUSH	JRN	13	0	(614)426-6185
TONDEB	TONEY,DEBRA	JRN	6	0	(513)828-1306

Total Number of Patients Listed: 13

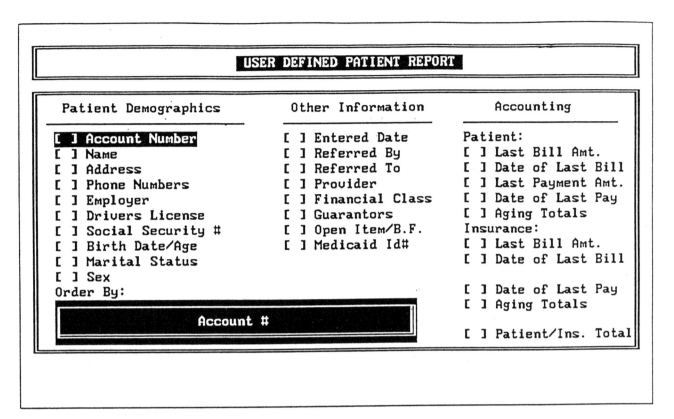

```
╔═══════════════════════════════════════════════════════════════════╗
║ ┌───────────────────────────────────────────────────────────────┐ ║
║ │              ▐ USER DEFINED PATIENT REPORT ▌                   │ ║
║ └───────────────────────────────────────────────────────────────┘ ║
║                                                                   ║
║   Patient Demographics      Other Information      Accounting      ║
║   ─────────────────────     ─────────────────     ──────────      ║
║   ▐ ] Account Number ▌      [ ] Entered Date     Patient:         ║
║   [ ] Name                  [ ] Referred By       [ ] Last Bill Amt. ║
║   [ ] Address               [ ] Referred To       [ ] Date of Last Bill ║
║   [ ] Phone Numbers         [ ] Provider          [ ] Last Payment Amt. ║
║   [ ] Employer              [ ] Financial Class   [ ] Date of Last Pay ║
║   [ ] Drivers License       [ ] Guarantors        [ ] Aging Totals ║
║   [ ] Social Security #     [ ] Open Item/B.F.   Insurance:       ║
║   [ ] Birth Date/Age        [ ] Medicaid Id#      [ ] Last Bill Amt. ║
║   [ ] Marital Status                              [ ] Date of Last Bill ║
║   [ ] Sex                                                          ║
║   Order By:                                        [ ] Date of Last Pay ║
║   ┌─────────────────────────────────────────┐     [ ] Aging Totals ║
║   │                Account #                │                     ║
║   └─────────────────────────────────────────┘     [ ] Patient/Ins. Total ║
╚═══════════════════════════════════════════════════════════════════╝
```

User Defined Patient Report Criteria Screen

The User Defined Patient Report is a report that you gives you only the information you specify. All aspects of a patient's data are available to you. You just check the boxes of the information you want on the report and just information will print.

You can also order this report in any order you want, there are over 50 choices for ordering your report these range from account # to patient and insurance balance.

Example Shown: User Defined Patient Report showing Account#, Name, and date of entry.

Account #: BURAMA
  Last Name: BURCHNELL   First Name: AMANDA   M.I.:L
Date of Entry:

Account #: CREHAU
  Last Name: CREAMER   First Name: HAUNS   M.I.:S
Date of Entry:

Account #: DAVJON
  Last Name: DAVIS   First Name: JONATHAN   M.I.:
Date of Entry:

Account #: DAVMAR
  Last Name: DAVIS   First Name: MARY   M.I.:L
Date of Entry:

Account #: ELLDOR
  Last Name: ELLIS   First Name: DOROTHY   M.I.:M
Date of Entry:

Account #: FREDAW
  Last Name: FREW   First Name: DAWN   M.I.:R
Date of Entry:

Account #: GRABET
  Last Name: GRAY   First Name: BETTY   M.I.:J
Date of Entry:

Account #: HENWES
  Last Name: HENDERSON   First Name: WESLEY   M.I.:M
Date of Entry:

Account #: LAWWIL
  Last Name: LAWSON   First Name: WILLIAM   M.I.:C
Date of Entry:

Account #: LEWTER
  Last Name: LEWIS   First Name: TERESA   M.I.:R
Date of Entry:

Account #: MONREE
  Last Name: MONROE   First Name: REED   M.I.:M
Date of Entry:

Account #: SHIRUS
  Last Name: SHIPE   First Name: RUSH   M.I.:R
Date of Entry:

Account #: TONDEB
  Last Name: TONEY   First Name: DEBRA   M.I.:L
Date of Entry:

Account #:
  Last Name: First Name: M.I.:
Date of Entry: / /

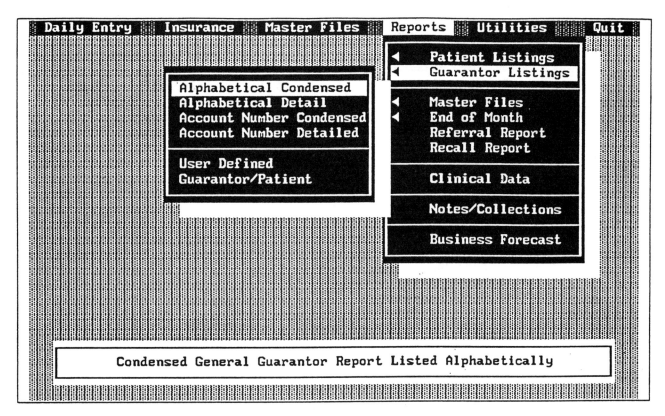

| Daily Entry | Insurance | Master Files | Reports | Utilities | Quit |

◄ Patient Listings
◄ Guarantor Listings

Alphabetical Condensed
Alphabetical Detail
Account Number Condensed
Account Number Detailed

User Defined
Guarantor/Patient

◄ Master Files
◄ End of Month
  Referral Report
  Recall Report

Clinical Data

Notes/Collections

Business Forecast

Condensed General Guarantor Report Listed Alphabetically

Screen Showing General Guarantor Listings

This is the main menu for the Guarantor Report section. These menu selections include general guarantor listings both in condensed and detailed formats, the guarantor grouping report and the guarantor user defined report. The guarantor/patient report which lists the guarantors and their related patients is also accessed from here.

Reports Shown on the following Pages:

User Defined Guarantor Report

107

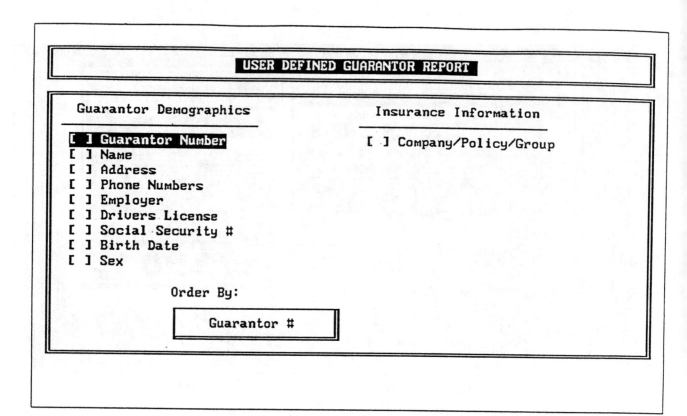

```
┌─────────────────────────────────────────────────────────────┐
│  ┌──────────────────────────────────────────────────────┐   │
│  │          USER DEFINED GUARANTOR REPORT               │   │
│  └──────────────────────────────────────────────────────┘   │
│  ┌──────────────────────────────────────────────────────┐   │
│  │  Guarantor Demographics      Insurance Information    │   │
│  │  ─────────────────────       ────────────────────     │   │
│  │  [ ] Guarantor Number        [ ] Company/Policy/Group │   │
│  │  [ ] Name                                             │   │
│  │  [ ] Address                                          │   │
│  │  [ ] Phone Numbers                                    │   │
│  │  [ ] Employer                                         │   │
│  │  [ ] Drivers License                                  │   │
│  │  [ ] Social Security #                                │   │
│  │  [ ] Birth Date                                       │   │
│  │  [ ] Sex                                              │   │
│  │                                                       │   │
│  │           Order By:                                   │   │
│  │         ┌──────────────────┐                         │   │
│  │         │   Guarantor #    │                         │   │
│  │         └──────────────────┘                         │   │
│  └──────────────────────────────────────────────────────┘   │
└─────────────────────────────────────────────────────────────┘
```

User Defined Guarantor Report

The User Defined Guarantor Report is a report that you gives you only the information you specify. All aspects of a guarantor's data are available to you. You just check the boxes of the information you want on the report and just that information will print.
You can also order this report in any order you want, there are over 25 choices for ordering you report these range from guarantor # to the guarantor's group #.

Example Shown: User Defined Guarantor Report showing guarantor #, name and social security #.

Guarantor #:   1
   Last Name: DAVIS   First Name: DONALD   M.I.:E
Social Security #: 287-32-2297

Guarantor #:   2
   Last Name: FREW   First Name: DAWN   M.I.:R
Social Security #: 275-72-5902

Guarantor #:   3
   Last Name: LAWSON   First Name: WILLIAM   M.I.:C
Social Security #: 273-20-5592

Guarantor #:   4
   Last Name: EVANS   First Name: ROGER   M.I.:D
Social Security #: 278-48-3205

Guarantor #:   5
   Last Name: ELLIS   First Name: DOROTHY   M.I.:M
Social Security #: 275-24-1903

Guarantor #:   6
   Last Name: TONEY   First Name: CURTIS   M.I.:R
Social Security #: 293-78-4553

Guarantor #:   7
   Last Name: CREAMER   First Name: STEVEN   M.I.:L
Social Security #: 274-64-3963

Guarantor #:   8
   Last Name: GRUBB   First Name: WANDA   M.I.:J
Social Security #: 275-66-6321

Guarantor #:   9
   Last Name: DAVIS   First Name: MARILYN   M.I.:K
Social Security #: 278-52-8167

Guarantor #:   10
   Last Name: BRIGGS   First Name: SHARON   M.I.:A
Social Security #: 296-82-9352

Guarantor #:   0
   Last Name: First Name: M.I.:
Social Security #:
      Total Number of Guarantors :   10

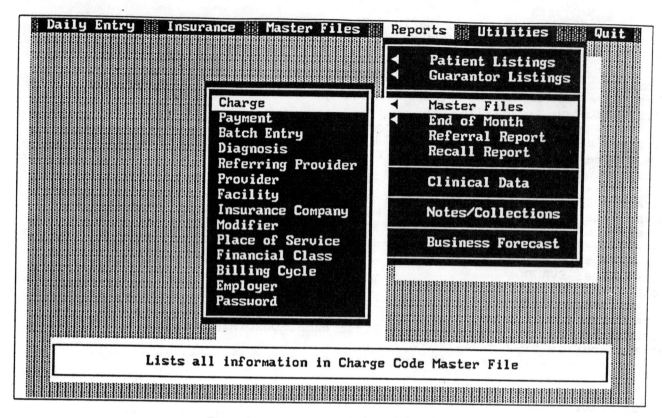

| Daily Entry | Insurance | Master Files | Reports | Utilities | Quit |

◄ Patient Listings
◄ Guarantor Listings

Charge
Payment
Batch Entry
Diagnosis
Referring Provider
Provider
Facility
Insurance Company
Modifier
Place of Service
Financial Class
Billing Cycle
Employer
Password

◄ Master Files
◄ End of Month
Referral Report
Recall Report

Clinical Data

Notes/Collections

Business Forecast

Lists all information in Charge Code Master File

Reports to List All Master Files

This is the main menu for the Master File Reports. There is a menu selection for each master file in Patriot Medical. These are complete listings of all the information you have in your master files. These are useful for desk side references.

Reports Shown of the following Pages:

None

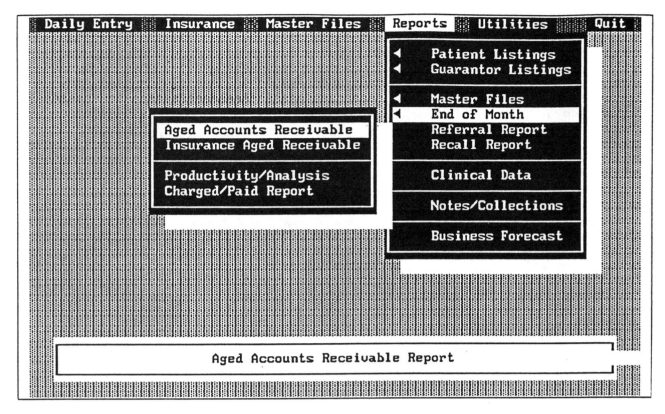

| Daily Entry | Insurance | Master Files | Reports | Utilities | Quit |

◄ Patient Listings
◄ Guarantor Listings

◄ Master Files
◄ End of Month
Referral Report
Recall Report

Aged Accounts Receivable
Insurance Aged Receivable

Productivity/Analysis
Charged/Paid Report

Clinical Data

Notes/Collections

Business Forecast

Aged Accounts Receivable Report

End of Month Reports

This is the main menu for the End of Month Reports. This lists the reports that we recommend be run on a monthly basis. These are mainly financial reports.
These include the aged accounts receivable report, the insurance aged accounts receivable report, the productivity/analysis report and the charge/paid report.

Reports Shown on the following pages:

Aged Accounts Receivable
Insurance Aged Receivable
Procedure Productivity Report
Charge/Paid Report

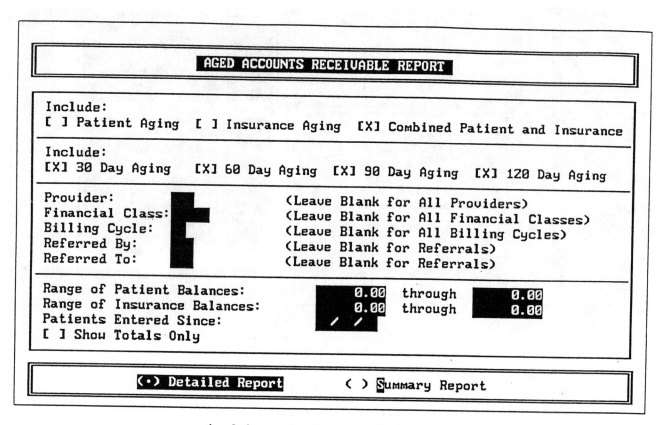

```
┌─────────────────────────────────────────────────────────────────┐
│ ┌─────────────────────────────────────────────────────────────┐ │
│ │          AGED ACCOUNTS RECEIVABLE REPORT                     │ │
│ └─────────────────────────────────────────────────────────────┘ │
│ ┌─────────────────────────────────────────────────────────────┐ │
│ │ Include:                                                      │ │
│ │ [ ] Patient Aging  [ ] Insurance Aging  [X] Combined Patient and Insurance │ │
│ │───────────────────────────────────────────────────────────── │ │
│ │ Include:                                                      │ │
│ │ [X] 30 Day Aging   [X] 60 Day Aging  [X] 90 Day Aging  [X] 120 Day Aging │ │
│ │───────────────────────────────────────────────────────────── │ │
│ │ Provider:          (Leave Blank for All Providers)           │ │
│ │ Financial Class:   (Leave Blank for All Financial Classes)   │ │
│ │ Billing Cycle:     (Leave Blank for All Billing Cycles)      │ │
│ │ Referred By:       (Leave Blank for Referrals)               │ │
│ │ Referred To:       (Leave Blank for Referrals)               │ │
│ │───────────────────────────────────────────────────────────── │ │
│ │ Range of Patient Balances:      0.00  through     0.00       │ │
│ │ Range of Insurance Balances:    0.00  through     0.00       │ │
│ │ Patients Entered Since:          / /                         │ │
│ │ [ ] Show Totals Only                                         │ │
│ └─────────────────────────────────────────────────────────────┘ │
│ ┌─────────────────────────────────────────────────────────────┐ │
│ │     (•) Detailed Report        ( ) Summary Report            │ │
│ └─────────────────────────────────────────────────────────────┘ │
└─────────────────────────────────────────────────────────────────┘
```

Aged Accounts Receivable Report

The Aged Accounts Receivable Report is part of the End of Month Reports. This lists your accounts receivable broken down into 30,60,90 and 120 day categories. This report is essential to tracking the financial health of your business.

This report has multiple criteria. It can be printed for patient, insurance and/or combined balances. You can isolate the report to one specific aging category as well. The report can be run for one particular provider or for the whole practice. Other criteria available is financial class, billing cycle, referred by, referred to. You may isolate patients with a range of insurance or patient balances. Lastly you can isolate patients by the date they were entered into the computer. The Aged Accounts Receivable report can be run in summary or detail. The summary listing lists each patient on one line giving you the 30,60,90 and 120 day breakdown and the total for the account. The detailed listing lists each patient with the same information as the summary plus the patients phone number, amount and date of last payment.

Example Shown: Summary Aged Accounts Receivable

112

****

Account #	Patient Name	Current	30	60	90	120	Total
BURAMA	BURCHNELL, AMANDA	0	360	0	0	0	360.00
CREHAU	CREAMER, HAUNS	0	0	0	0	0	0.00
DAVJON	DAVIS, JONATHAN	0	360	0	0	0	360.00
DAVMAR	DAVIS, MARY	0	147	0	0	0	147.00
ELLDOR	ELLIS, DOROTHY	0	270	0	0	0	270.00
FREDAW	FREW, DAWN	0	450	0	0	0	450.00
GRABET	GRAY, BETTY	0	2835	0	0	0	2835.00
HENWES	HENDERSON, WESLEY	0	315	0	0	0	315.00
LAWWIL	LAWSON, WILLIAM	0	1080	0	0	0	1080.00
LEWTER	LEWIS, TERESA	0	24	0	0	0	24.00
MONREE	MONROE, REED	0	450	0	0	0	450.00
SHIRUS	SHIPE, RUSH	0	540	0	0	0	450.00
TONDEB	TONEY, DEBRA	0	495	0	0	0	495.00

Grand Totals:

	Current	30	60	90	120	Total
Patient:	0.00	171.00	0.00	0.00	0.00	171.00
Insurance:	0.00	7155.00	0.00	0.00	0.00	7155.00

| | 0.00 | 7326.00 | 0.00 | 0.00 | 0.00 | 7326.00 |

113

```
┌─────────────────────────────────────────────────────────────────────────┐
│  ┌───────────────────────────────────────────────────────────────────┐  │
│  │              INSURANCE AGED RECEIVABLE REPORT                       │  │
│  └───────────────────────────────────────────────────────────────────┘  │
│                                                                           │
│  Account #: ▉▉▉▉▉▉▉      Range( ▉▉▉▉▉▉▉▉    through ▉▉▉▉ ▉▉ )             │
│                         (Leave Blank for all Accounts)                    │
│  ───────────────────────────────────────────────────────────────────     │
│  Provider Code: ▉▉      Range( ▉▉ through ▉▉ )                            │
│                         (Leave Blank for all Providers)                   │
│  ───────────────────────────────────────────────────────────────────     │
│  Insurance Company Code: ▉▉▉▉▉▉   Range( ▉▉▉▉▉▉▉   through ▉▉▉▉▉ )        │
│                         (Leave Blank for all Insurance Companies)         │
│  ───────────────────────────────────────────────────────────────────     │
│  Insurance Form Amount: ▉▉0.00 Range( ▉▉▉0.00 through ▉▉▉0.0 )           │
│                         (Leave Blank for all Insurance Form Amounts)      │
│  ───────────────────────────────────────────────────────────────────     │
│  Insurance Filed Date: ▉ / / ▉   Range( ▉ / / ▉ through ▉ / / ▉ )        │
│                         (Leave Blank for all Insurance Form Filed Dates)  │
│  ───────────────────────────────────────────────────────────────────     │
│  Print Status: ▉▉▉▉▉▉    (NOT PRNTD/PRNTD)   Leave Blank for all Forms    │
│                                                                           │
│  ┌───────────────────────────────────────────────────────────────────┐  │
│  │   (•) Summary Listing      ( ) Detailed Listing                    │  │
│  └───────────────────────────────────────────────────────────────────┘  │
└─────────────────────────────────────────────────────────────────────────┘
```

Insurance Aged Accounts Receivable Criteria Screen

The Insurance Aged Accounts Receivable Report is part of the End of Month Reports. This lists your insurance form aging broken down by Insurance Company. This report is essential in tracking the payment of your claims.

The report has multiple criteria. It can be printed for one account or a range of accounts, one provider or a range of providers, one insurance company or a range of companies, one dollar amount or range of dollar amounts, one filed date or a range of dates filed as well by the print status of the claim.

The Insurance Aged Receivable report can be run in summary or detail. The summary report shows the insurance company name, phone number and contact. The total aging broken down into 30,60,90 and 120 days is listed. The detail report lists each insurance company as in the summary report in addition each insurance form is listed on one line represented by an Account#, Form #, Date Filed and the form amount. A total is at the end of the report also breaking down the percentage of each category.

Example Shown: Detailed Insurance Aging Report

Condensed Insurance Aging Report Based on Insurance Filed Date

Current	>30	>60	>90	>120	Total

`*****************************************************************************`

BLUE   Blue Cross (419)874-0162/   Contact: Polly Bart Remark: BENEFITS

Account #	Form #	Date Filed	Amount
DANBET	19	08/31/	60.00
DANBET	22	08/31/	140.00
DANBET	23	08/31/	840.00
DANBET	24	08/31/	4750.00
DANBET	25	09/18/	6650.00
DANBET	26	09/18/	200.00
DANBET	27	09/18/	399.90
NICJAC	18	06/22/	125.00

Current	>30	>60	>90	>120	Total
0.00	0.00	0.00	0.00	13164.90	13164.90

CIGNA   Cigna Life (916)889-1212/   Contact: Bertha Ski Remark:

Account #	Form #	Date Filed	Amount
DOWJEA	20	08/31/	60.00

Current	>30	>60	>90	>120	Total
0.00	0.00	0.00	0.00	60.00	60.00

PRUDENTIAL Prudential (092)480-2349/82308 Contact: MARLA THOM Remark: 234092

Account #	Form #	Date Filed	Amount
DAVFRA	2	05/21/	395.00
DAVFRA	3	05/21/	450.00
DAVFRA	4	07/06/	225.00
DAVFRA	16	06/12/	150.00
DAVFRA	17	06/15/	75.00
FOXTIF	5	05/21/	20.00
FOXWIL03	6	06/01/	55.00
FOXWIL03	7	06/01/	0.00
FOXWIL03	8	06/01/	0.00
FOXWIL03	9	06/01/	0.00
FOXWIL03	10	06/01/	55.00
FOXWIL03	11	06/05/	205.00
FOXWIL03	12	06/05/	75.00
FOXWIL03	15	06/05/	75.00

Current	>30	>60	>90	>120	Total
0.00	0.00	0.00	0.00	1780.00	1780.00

Totals: `***********************************************************`

Current	>30	>60	>90	>120	Total
0.00	0.00	0.00	0.00	15004.90	15004.90

Percent of Total Aged: `*********************************************`

Current	>30	>60	>90	>120	
0.00	0.00	0.00	0.00	100.00	

```
┌─────────────────────────────────────────────────────────────────────────┐
│  ┌───────────────────────────────────────────────────────────────────┐  │
│  │            ▐PROCEDURE/DX ANALYSIS/PRODUCTIVITY▌                     │  │
│  └───────────────────────────────────────────────────────────────────┘  │
│  ┌───────────────────────────────────────────────────────────────────┐  │
│  │              Procedure Code Productivity Report                    │  │
│  │                                                                   │  │
│  │  Procedure Code:    ████████      Range(███████  Through ████████  │  │
│  │                        (Leave Blank for All Codes)                │  │
│  │  User Code:         ████████      Range( █████  Through  ██████ )  │  │
│  │                        (Leave Blank for All Codes)                │  │
│  │  Transaction Date:  ██/ /██      Range( ██/ /██ Through ██/ /██ )  │  │
│  │                   (Leave Blank for All Transaction Dates)         │  │
│  ├───────────────────────────────────────────────────────────────────┤  │
│  │  Provider Code:             █      Range(█    Through       )      │  │
│  │  Place of Service Code:     █      Range(█    Through       )      │  │
│  │  Financial Class:           █      Range(█    Through       )      │  │
│  │  Type of Service Code:      █      Range(█    Through  ·    )      │  │
│  │                                                                   │  │
│  │  [ ] Show Totals Only     Subtotal Report By:  ▐Provider/Account #▌│  │
│  └───────────────────────────────────────────────────────────────────┘  │
│  ┌───────────────────────────────────────────────────────────────────┐  │
│  │    ▐(·) Detailed Listing▌       ( ) Summary Listing               │  │
│  └───────────────────────────────────────────────────────────────────┘  │
└─────────────────────────────────────────────────────────────────────────┘
```

Procedure/Dx Productivity and/or Analysis Report

The Procedure/Dx Analysis Report is three types of reports in one. You may print a Productivity Procedure Report, Productivity Analysis Report and Diagnosis Productivity Report. The report is designed to give you information on the volume of procedures you are performing plus the amount of adjustments you are making and the amount of money you are collecting.

The productivity report has multiple choices in the order you want the report listed. You may order the report by provider and then by account#, place of service and account#, financial class and then by account #, procedure code, type of service and then account#, provider and then type of service, place of service then type of service, lastly diagnosis. Depending on the list you choose the information will be displayed differently.

This report listing can be run in summary or detail. The summary option lists totals for each procedure code. The detail report lists each code and each transaction that falls under the procedure, adjustment or payment code.

Example Shown: Detailed Procedure Productivity listed by Procedure Code.

Code	Account#	Patient	Date	Dx Code	Units	Charge

****

Type of Service: 7
00120   ANESTHESIA FOR EAR SURGERY

T/T	BURAMA	BURCHNELL,AMAND	01/05/	381.10	8	45.00
	CREHAU	CREAMER,HAUNS	01/05/	381.10	8	45.00
	HENWES	HENDERSON,WESLE	01/05/	478.0	7	45.00

					23	1035.00

00160   ANESTH pro on nose and acc sinuses not s

	DAVJON	DAVIS,JONATHAN	01/05/	478.0	8	45.00

					8	360.00

00170   ANESTH intraoral pro incl biopsy not s

T/A	TONDEB	TONEY,DEBRA	01/05/	474.0	11	45.00

					11	495.00

00860   ANESTH extraper in low abd inc urinary t

	FREDAW	FREW,DAWN	01/04/	592.1	10	45.00

					10	450.00

01382   ANESTH arthroscopic pro of knee joint

	DAVMAR	DAVIS,MARY	01/04/	715.16	11	45.00

					11	495.00

62274   INJECT SPINAL ANESTHETIC

SPINAL	LEWTER	LEWIS,TERESA	01/04/	650.	8	45.00

					8	360.00

*** TOTALS ***   Payments: 0   0.00 Charges: 71   3195.00

```
┌──────────────────────────────────────────────────────────────────────────┐
│ ┌────────────────────────────────────────────────────────────────────────┐ │
│ │                     █ CHARGED/PAID REPORT █                              │ │
│ └────────────────────────────────────────────────────────────────────────┘ │
│ ┌────────────────────────────────────────────────────────────────────────┐ │
│ │ Charge Code:          ████    Range( ████   through ████ )              │ │
│ │                 (Leave Blank for All Charge Codes)                       │ │
│ │                                                                          │ │
│ │ Date of Service for Charge: ██/██  Range( ██/██ through ██/██ )         │ │
│ │             Leave Blank to Report Regardless of Date of Service          │ │
│ ├────────────────────────────────────────────────────────────────────────┤ │
│ │             (Leave Options Blank to Include All Items)                   │ │
│ │ Account #:         ████    Range( ████        through ████ )            │ │
│ │ Insurance Company Code: ████   Range( ████    through ████ )            │ │
│ │ Financial Class:   ████    Range( ██ through ██ )                       │ │
│ │ Provider Code:     ████    Range( ██ through ██ )                       │ │
│ ├────────────────────────────────────────────────────────────────────────┤ │
│ │ Subtotal Report By:                                                      │ │
│ │                    ┌─────────────────────────┐                          │ │
│ │                    │      Charge Code         │                          │ │
│ │                    └─────────────────────────┘                          │ │
│ └────────────────────────────────────────────────────────────────────────┘ │
│ ┌────────────────────────────────────────────────────────────────────────┐ │
│ │  █(•) Detailed Listing█    ( ) §ummary Listing    ( ) ⛶otal Only        │ │
│ └────────────────────────────────────────────────────────────────────────┘ │
└──────────────────────────────────────────────────────────────────────────┘
```

Charge/Paid Criteria Screen

The Charge/Paid Report is part of the End of Month Reports. This sophisticated report is essential in tracking your reimbursement rates from HMO's, PPO's and any other carriers you submit to. In addition, how much you are receiving from your different payment sources (patient, insurance and write off's) in dollars and percentages.

This report can be isolated by one charge code or a range of codes, one date of service or a range of dates of service, one account number or a range, one insurance company or a range, one financial class or a range, one provider or range. The report can be subtotaled by charge code, account #, insurance company, or provider code.

The summary report gives you a total for all activity defined by your criteria specifications. The detailed report breaks down the report by code and gives you totals for each procedure code.

The report lists the amounts allowed by insurance companies for each charge, the amount you are actually collecting from the insurance company, the amount you are collecting from the patients. The percentages are broken down so that you can see the percentage of collected amounts from these different sources.

Example Shown: Summary Charge/Paid Report

Summary Charge/Paid Report
Subtotal By: Charge Code

Total Charges in Range	Charges w/Payments & W/O in R	Patient Payments Applied	Insurance Payments Applied	Write Off's Applied in Range	Allowed Total in Range	% of Allowed Paid by Insurance
****

62278   EPIDURAL INJECTION, SINGLE

| 62.03 | 62.03 | 12.41 | 49.62 | 0.00 | 50.00 | 99.24 |
| % of Charged in Range: | | 20.01 | 79.99 | 0.00 | | |

81000   URINALYSIS

| 420.00 | 420.00 | 0.00 | 20.00 | 20.00 | 320.00 | 6.25 |
| % of Charged in Range: | | 0.00 | 4.76 | 4.76 | | |

90050   REGULAR OFFICE VISIT

| 350.00 | 350.00 | 76.00 | 162.00 | 131.00 | 294.00 | 55.10 |
| % of Charged in Range: | | 21.71 | 46.29 | 37.43 | | |

TOTALS: ***

| 832.03 | 832.03 | 88.41 | 231.62 | 151.00 | 34.88 | 53.53 |
| | | 20.86 | 43.68 | 21.10 | | |

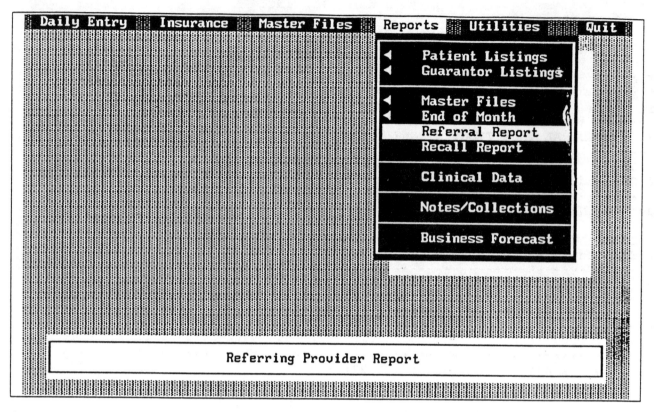

| Daily Entry | Insurance | Master Files | Reports | Utilities | Quit |

◄ Patient Listings
◄ Guarantor Listings

◄ Master Files
◄ End of Month
Referral Report
Recall Report

Clinical Data

Notes/Collections

Business Forecast

Referring Provider Report

Main Report Menu Showing Other Reports Available

This is the main reports menu, menus for patient, guarantor, master files and end of month reports are accessed from here. In addition other reports are accessed directly from this menu. These include the Referral Report, Recall Report, Clinical Data Report, Notes/Collections and the Business Forecast Report.

Reports Shown on the following pages:

Referral Report
Recall Report
Clinical Data Report
Notes/Collections Report
Business Status and Forecast Report

```
┌──────────────────────────────────────────────────────────────────┐
│  ┌──────────────────────────────────────────────────────────────┐ │
│  │              ▐ RERERRING PROVIDER REPORT ▌                     │ │
│  └──────────────────────────────────────────────────────────────┘ │
│ ┌────────────────────────────────────────────────────────────────┐│
│ │ Referring Provider Code: ▐▌        Range( ▐▌ Through ▐▌ )       ││
│ ├────────────────────────────────────────────────────────────────┤│
│ │ Patient Entry Date:    From ▐ / / ▌  Through ▐ / / ▌            ││
│ │                  (Leave Blank for All Entry Dates)             ││
│ │                                                                ││
│ │                         ✶✶✶ OR ✶✶✶                            ││
│ │                                                                ││
│ │ Transaction Entry Date: From ▐ / / ▌  Through ▐ / / ▌          ││
│ │                  (Leave Blank for All Transaction Dates)       ││
│ ├────────────────────────────────────────────────────────────────┤│
│ │ Include Patient Detail:     N                                  ││
│ │                                                                ││
│ │ Include Transaction Detail: N                                  ││
│ └────────────────────────────────────────────────────────────────┘│
│                                                                    │
│             To Report on One Referring Provider                    │
└──────────────────────────────────────────────────────────────────┘
```

Referring Provider Report

The Referring Provider Report keeps track of the patients that were referred to you by other sources. It can be used to keep track of referring physicians, advertisements or other referring sources. Depending on your specialty this information can be critical to your business. You can now track who is sending you what and how much income each resource is generating for you. This report has several criteria options, you can print the report for one referring source or a range. The report can be isolated to patients that were entered in your computer in range of dates, you can also isolate patients by the date of transaction. Depending on the amount of detail you require you may include the actual patient detail and/or transaction detail.

Example Shown: Referring Provider Report Showing Patient Detail

```
ame:
 ccount#        Entered       Charges      Payments  Adjustments     Balance
*****************************************************************************
 rovider: ETA  Name: Edward T. Arcy D.O.           Phone: (614)889-8900
 AVMAR        01/15/         495.00        0.00         0.00         495.00
 FREDAW       01/15/         450.00        0.00         0.00         450.00
 EWTER        01/15/         360.00        0.00         0.00         360.00
 ONDEB        01/16/         495.00        0.00         0.00         495.00

 ---------------------------------------------------------------------------
 :    4   ** TOTAL ***      1800.00        0.00         0.00        1800.00
 ---------------------------------------------------------------------------

 rovider: ETA  Name: Kirk W. Schnoeman D.C.         Phone:
 URAMA        01/16/         360.00        0.00         0.00         360.00
 CREHAU       01/16/         360.00        0.00         0.00         360.00
 DAVJON       01/16/         360.00        0.00         0.00         360.00
 ENWES        01/16/         315.00        0.00         0.00         315.00

 ---------------------------------------------------------------------------
 :    4   ** TOTAL ***      1395.00        0.00         0.00        1395.00
 ---------------------------------------------------------------------------
```

```
┌─────────────────────────────────────────────────────────────────┐
│  ╔═══════════════════════════════════════════════════════════╗  │
│  ║              PATIENT RECALL REPORT                        ║  │
│  ╚═══════════════════════════════════════════════════════════╝  │
│                                                                   │
│  Recall Date: ▓ / / ▓        Range( ▓ / / ▓ Through ▓ / / ▓ )    │
│                     (Leave Blank for Dates)                       │
│  ───────────────────────────────────────────────────────────────│
│  Reason Code: ▓▓▓▓         Range( ▓▓▓ Through ▓▓▓ )              │
│                   (Leave Blank for Reason Codes)                  │
│  ───────────────────────────────────────────────────────────────│
│  Account #:  ▓▓▓▓▓▓       Range( ▓▓▓▓▓ Through ▓▓▓▓▓ )           │
│                   (Leave Blank for All Accounts)                  │
│  ───────────────────────────────────────────────────────────────│
│  Provider Code:   ▓       Range( ▓    Through    )               │
│  Financial Class: ▓       Range( ▓    Through    )               │
│  Birth Date:    ▓ / / ▓   Range( ▓ / / ▓ Through ▓ / / ▓ )       │
│  ───────────────────────────────────────────────────────────────│
│  Patient Entry Date: ▓ / / ▓  Range( ▓ / / ▓ Through ▓ / / ▓ )   │
│                                                                   │
│                                                                   │
│                   To Report on One Recall Date                    │
└─────────────────────────────────────────────────────────────────┘
```

Patient Recall Report

The Patient Recall Report is used to list your patients that you have set up for recall. Recall allows you to set up patients to be recalled at a certain time and for a certain reason.

The Recall Report can be printed using several criteria options, the recall date or a range of dates, a reason or a range of reason codes, one account # or a range of account #'s, a provider code or a range of provider codes, a financial class or a range of classes, a birth date or a range of birth dates, lastly, a date the patient was entered into the computer or a range of dates.

The Recall Report groups patients by the recall date and lists the patient account #, the patient first and last name, the patients phone #, their primary provider, the time they are scheduled to come in and the reason. In addition the patient & insurance balances and the date of last payment. Finally the patients account balance is listed.

Example Shown: Patient Recall Report

SMITH & KLINE MD, INC.

Patient Recall Report

```
Account #    Name            Phone/Ext           Pr  Time  Reason
*****************************************************************************
Recall Date: 03/23/
*********************
GRABET      GRAY,BETTY       (614)869-4100/      JRN  10:00 90220  Admission
Balance Patient:      0.00  DOL:  / /   Insurance:  2835.00  DOL:   / /
Account Balance:   2835.00
-----------------------------------------------------------------------------

-----------------------------------------------------------------------------


Recall Date: 03/28/
*********************
CREHAU      CREAMER,HAUNS    (614)852-0229/      JRN  12:50 99070  Upper Arm
Balance Patient:      0.00  DOL: 02/28/93  Insurance:     0.00  DOL: 02/04/93
Account Balance:      0.00
-----------------------------------------------------------------------------
BURAMA      BURCHNELL,AMAND (614)852-4951/      JRN  12:00 99070  Upper Arm
Balance Patient:      0.00  DOL:  / /   Insurance:   360.00  DOL:   / /
Account Balance:    360.00
-----------------------------------------------------------------------------

-----------------------------------------------------------------------------
```

```
┌─────────────────────────────────────────────────────────────────────┐
│  ┌───────────────────────────────────────────────────────────────┐   │
│  │                  PATIENT CLINICAL DATA REPORT                 │   │
│  └───────────────────────────────────────────────────────────────┘   │
│  ┌───────────────────────────────────────────────────────────────┐   │
│  │  Account #: ▓▓▓▓▓▓▓     Range( ▓▓▓▓▓▓ through ▓▓▓▓▓▓ )        │   │
│  │              (Leave Blank for all Accounts)                    │   │
│  ├───────────────────────────────────────────────────────────────┤   │
│  │  Provider Code: ▓▓     Range( ▓▓ through ▓▓ )                 │   │
│  │              (Leave Blank for all Providers)                   │   │
│  ├───────────────────────────────────────────────────────────────┤   │
│  │  Diagnosis Code: ▓▓▓▓    Range( ▓▓▓▓ through ▓▓▓▓ )           │   │
│  │              (Leave Blank for all Diagnosis Codes)             │   │
│  ├───────────────────────────────────────────────────────────────┤   │
│  │  Date: ▓ / / ▓    Range( ▓ / / ▓ through ▓ / / ▓ )           │   │
│  │              (Leave Blank for all Dates                        │   │
│  ├───────────────────────────────────────────────────────────────┤   │
│  │  Referred By: ▓    Range( ▓ through ▓ )                       │   │
│  │  Referred To: ▓    Range( ▓ through ▓ )                       │   │
│  │  Active Patient:▓                                              │   │
│  │  Sex:▓   Age: ▓    Zip Code: ▓▓▓▓▓▓                           │   │
│  └───────────────────────────────────────────────────────────────┘   │
└─────────────────────────────────────────────────────────────────────┘
```

Clinical Data Report Criteria Screen

The Patient Clinical Data Report lists the clinical data you have on file for your patients. This includes chronic diagnoses, medications, allergies, clinical alert, age, sex and referring physician. This report has several criteria options for you to isolate your listing in to the group of patients you are interested in. The report can be printed for one account or a range of accounts, one provider or a range of providers, one diagnosis code or a range of codes, one date or a range of dates, one referring physician or a range of referring physicians, one referred to physician or a range of refereed to physicians. You may base the report on active patients, a patient's sex and/or a patients particular zip code.

If you are looking for a group of patients that have been diagnosed with a certain diagnosis this report will give you that information.

Example Shown: Patient Clinical Data Report

Patient Clincal Data Report

Account #	Name:	Provider	Age	Sex	Zip	Active

CREHAU   CREAMER, HAUNS   JRN   M   43140
           Referred By: KWS   Kirk W. Schn
           Dx Code: 487   INFLUENZA

MONREE   MONROE, REED   JRN   M   45368   Y
           Dx Code: 491.0   SIMPLE CHRONIC BRONCHITIS

SHIRUS   SHIPE, RUSH   JRN   M   43128   Y
           Dx Code: 701.1   KERATODERMA

```
┌──────────────────────────────────────────────────────────────────┐
│  ┌──────────────────────────────────────────────────────────┐     │
│  │            PATIENT NOTES/COLLECTION REPORT                │     │
│  └──────────────────────────────────────────────────────────┘     │
│  ┌──────────────────────────────────────────────────────────┐     │
│  │  Entry User Code:▓▓▓        [ ] All Patients             │     │
│  │                                                            │     │
│  │  Tickle Date:▓/ / ▓     Range(▓ / / ▓ through ▓ / / ▓    │     │
│  │                                                            │     │
│  │  Account #:  ▓▓▓▓▓▓    Range( ▓▓▓▓▓▓  through ▓▓▓▓▓▓ )    │     │
│  │              (Leave Blank for All Account #'s)            │     │
│  │                                                            │     │
│  │  Financial Class:▓▓▓   Range( ▓▓▓ through ▓▓▓ )          │     │
│  │            (Leave Blank for All Financial Classes         │     │
│  │                                                            │     │
│  │  Billing Cycle:  ▓     Range( ▓ through ▓)               │     │
│  │            (Leave Blank for All Billing Cycles            │     │
│  │                                                            │     │
│  │  Balance:  ▓ 0.00      Range( ▓ 0.00 through ▓ 0.00)     │     │
│  │            (Leave Blank for Patient Balances)            │     │
│  │  Aging: Cur:▓0.00 >30 ▓0.00 >60 ▓0.00 >90 ▓0.00>120 ▓0.00│     │
│  └──────────────────────────────────────────────────────────┘     │
│  ┌──────────────────────────────────────────────────────────┐     │
│  │    (•) Detailed Listing        ( ) Summary Listing       │     │
│  └──────────────────────────────────────────────────────────┘     │
└──────────────────────────────────────────────────────────────────┘
```

Patient Notes/Collections Report

The Patient Notes/Collection Report is a report designed to aide you in your collection process. All the information regarding a patient in terms of collections is present on this report.

The report is designed to be used in conjunction with your patient notes, however can also be used for patients that do not have notes on file. The notes allow you to keep a very close tab on your collection efforts.

The Patient Notes/Collection Report criteria screen presents you with several criteria options. The report is available in summary or detailed format. The summary report lists the patient account #, name, financial class, billing cycle, age, guarantors, guarantor's name, guarantor's employer and guarantor's/patient's insurance coverage. The detailed report gives you all the information in the summary option as well as the patient's insurance and patient balance information including aging. If there are any notes on file for the patient these are printed in both the summary and detailed options.

Example Shown: Detailed Patient Notes/Collection Report

Date:
Time:18:13:28

Patient Notes Report

```
.ccount #    Name:                      Financial Class  Billing Cycle   Age
*************************************************************************
1ONREE      MONROE,REED                 MCARE                5           76
 Ph #1: (513)462-8519/              Ph #2:            /
 Guarantor #1:     11 MONROE,REED  Employer:
 Insurance Code: MEDICARE   Nationwide Ins./Medicare Ops.
atient ==>
 Last Amt. Billed:      0.00 on  / /    Last Amt. Paid:     0.00 on  / /
 Aging: Cr:      0 >30       0 >60        0 >90      0 >120       0
Insurance ==>
 Last Amt. Billed:    450.00 on 02/28/93  Last Amt. Paid:    0.00 on  / /
 Aging.: Cr:      0 >30     450 >60        0 >90      0 >120       0
 Total:      0.00       450.00        0.00        0.00          0.00
 Balance:  Patient:      0.00  Insurance:   450.00  Account:    450.00
-----------------------------------------------------------------------
 Entry Date: 03/18/    Entry User: DMO Tickle Date: 03/28/
 Always forgets appts call before next appt to remind her
-----------------------------------------------------------------------
-----------------------------------------------------------------------
 Total Number of Notes on File for Account # MONREE:   1

 HIRUS      SHIPE,RUSH                  CIGNA                5           59
 Ph #1: (614)426-6185/              Ph #2:            /
 Guarantor #1:     13 SHIPE,RUSH  Employer:
 Insurance Code: CIGNA HEAL not found in Master File
atient ==>
 Last Amt. Billed:      0.00 on  / /    Last Amt. Paid:     0.00 on  / /
 Aging: Cr:      0 >30       0 >60        0 >90      0 >120       0
nsurance ==>
 Last Amt. Billed:    450.00 on 03/08/  Last Amt. Paid:     0.00 on  / /
 Aging.: Cr:      0 >30     540 >60        0 >90      0 >120       0
 Total:      0.00       540.00        0.00        0.00          0.00
 Balance:  Patient:      0.00  Insurance:   540.00  Account:    540.00
-----------------------------------------------------------------------
 Entry Date: 03/18/    Entry User: DMO Tickle Date:  / /
 Check current coverage not effective until 3/13/
-----------------------------------------------------------------------
 Total Number of Notes on File for Account # SHIRUS:   1
*************************************************************************
'otal Number of Patients Listed:   2
```

128

```
┌──────────────────────────────────────────────────────────────┐
│  ┌──────────────────────────────────────────────────────────┐ │
│  │           ██ BUSINESS STATUS AND FORECAST ██              │ │
│  └──────────────────────────────────────────────────────────┘ │
│  ┌════════════════════════Business Status On   /   / ═══════┐ │
│  │ Patient Billings:              Patient Payments:          │ │
│  │  MTD: 205.00      W/O: 0.00     MTD: 4987.49    W/O: 56.00 │ │
│  │  YTD: 205.00      W/O: 0.00     YTD: 4987.49    W/O: 56.00 │ │
│  │  Posted Today: 135.00           Posted Today: 360.00      │ │
│  │                                                           │ │
│  │ Insurance Billings:            Insurance Payments:        │ │
│  │  MTD: 200.00      W/O: 0.00     MTD: 210.00     W/O: 15.00 │ │
│  │  YTD: 200.00      W/O: 0.00     YTD: 210.00     W/O: 15.00 │ │
│  │  Posted Today: 1890.00          Posted Today: 2202.00     │ │
│  │                                                           │ │
│  │ Total Accounts Receivable: 61719.00                       │ │
│  │                                                           │ │
│  │ Number of Insurance Forms Outstanding: 23   Amount: 15004.90│ │
│  │                                                           │ │
│  │ Number of New Patients:   Today: 53   MTD: 75   YTD: 100  │ │
│  └───────────────────────────────────────────────────────────┘ │
│  ┌───────────────────────────────────────────────────────────┐ │
│  │  ██ ‹ › Forecast ██      ‹·› Return Without Forecasting    │ │
│  └───────────────────────────────────────────────────────────┘ │
└──────────────────────────────────────────────────────────────┘
```

Business Status Report

The Business Status and Forecast is unique to Patriot Medical. The business status report gives you the ability to see the current financial status of your practice with a touch of key and at any given time.

This report is a one screen picture of the financial status of your practice today. The patient and insurance billings are divided reporting daily, monthly and year to date breakdowns. The number of insurance forms and the dollar amount of those forms is listed as well. The number of new patients seen today, this month and this year is also listed.

Example Shown on this page: Business Status Report

```
┌─────────────────────────────────────────────────────────────┐
│  ┌─────────────────────────────────────────────────────────┐ │
│  │         ▐ BUSINESS STATUS AND FORECAST ▌                 │ │
│  └─────────────────────────────────────────────────────────┘ │
│  ┌──────────────════Business Forecast On 03/18/ ════────────┐ │
│  │ Patient Totals:        Current:          Projected:      │ │
│  │ ─────────────                                            │ │
│  │ Patient Billings:        205.00             861.00       │ │
│  │ Patient Payments:       4987.49           20947.46       │ │
│  │ Patient Debit W/O's:       0.00               0.00       │ │
│  │ Credit W/O's:             56.00             235.20       │ │
│  │─────────────────────────────────────────────────────────│ │
│  │ Insurance Totals:                                        │ │
│  │ ─────────────────                                        │ │
│  │ Insurance Billings:      200.00             840.00       │ │
│  │ Insurance Payments:      210.00             882.00       │ │
│  │ Insurance Debit W/O's:     0.00               0.00       │ │
│  │ Credit W/O's:             15.00              63.00       │ │
│  │─────────────────────────────────────────────────────────│ │
│  │ Accounts Receivable:   61719.00           46155.83       │ │
│  │ New Patients:             75                 315         │ │
│  └─────────────────────────────────────────────────────────┘ │
│  ┌─────────────────────────────────────────────────────────┐ │
│  │ ▐ < > Print Status and Forecast ▌   <·> ▐R▌eturn Without Printing │ │
│  └─────────────────────────────────────────────────────────┘ │
└─────────────────────────────────────────────────────────────┘
```

Business Forecast Report

The Forecast Report is based on the information compiled in the Business Status report. The forecast report predicts the future. The forecast is based on past performance.

The report will be able to determine you expected billings, payments, write offs/adjustments and accounts receivable. The forecast also calculates the number of patients you can expect to see. This report is based on the number of working days in the month and the number remaining.

Example Shown on this page: Business Forecast Report